Nubia's Guide to Going Natural

A Holistic Approach to Transitioning Your Hair

Orjanette Bryant

AuthorHouse™
1663 Liberty Drive
Bloomington, IN 47403
www.authorhouse.com
Phone: 1-800-839-8640

Published by AuthorHouse 04/01/2015

ISBN: 978-1-4969-5219-6 (sc)
ISBN: 978-1-4969-5220-2 (e)

Print information available on the last page.

http://commons.wikimedia.org/wiki/File%3AAvocado_open.jpg

http://pixabay.com/en/avocado-fruit-vegetable-green-seed-71567/

authorHOUSE®

CONTENTS

INTRODUCTION

With all the confusing information out there, I want to simplify and provide a reference to help you understand the best options to hair care without the harmful use of the chemicals we use daily. As a natural hair consultant, motivational speaker, and a nurse in the health care for over 20 years I educate others about preventive measures and help others understand how chemicals affect our wellbeing.

Although this book was intended primarily for African Americans wanting to go natural, some of this information is beneficial for everyone. People everywhere can benefit from the best hair care solutions. Growing our hair and improving our overall health is a shared interest. Transitioning to natural hair care strengthens you spiritually, physically, and emotionally.

There is a profound emotional effect that occurs when transitioning from chemically processed to natural hair. Most people who wear their hair natural begin to experience an increase in their self-esteem. I have personally noticed people exuding more confidence when they begin to wear their hair natural. I often hear people expressing that they are afraid to go natural. I remember feeling that way myself. I was once encouraged by a close friend to try going natural. She assured me that going natural is not complicated, and that she loved my natural hair. I vehemently responded that I would never go natural. I remember feeling afraid of the kinks and intimidated by the work required to manage my hair without a perm.

Some people transition to natural to improve their quality of life. I can attest to feeling mentally relieved and refreshed after transitioning from processed hair. The European look was not for me. I have learned to embrace my kinks and love my naps. As you embark and enjoy your natural hair journey you will become more confident about your new look. You will experience fewer headaches, infections, and less medical problems when you let go of the routine use of the harsh chemicals. I do not recall any warning labels informing those who use perms and other chemicals on their hair about the adverse effects of the products. My goal is to provide you with a wealth of knowledge that will help guide you along your transition to natural, thus enabling you to avoid the negative results of using harsh chemicals on your scalp. *Nubia's Guide to Going Natural* will help you understand your hair and types of chemicals that are highly recommended for the hair.

This guide offers valuable information and money savings tips, as you transition to natural, unprocessed hair. Going natural is important. There are some psychological aspects of going natural and you may find many social, mental, and behavioral benefits to wearing your hair natural. We often hear people saying, "I just can't wear my hair in its natural state". This book challenges your beliefs about the use of chemicals. Chemicals destroy or cause irreversible damage to your hair. You will learn how to transform your hair from nappy to happy through the use of organic products.

ACKNOWLEDGEMENTS

I want to thank my Lord and Savior for his inspiration in writing this book. To my husband Ron Bryant, my closest friend and inspiration and creator of Cut N Edge Cartoons, GG Comics, and the self—syndicated political cartoonist known as "Cut." I could not have done this book without the support of my family and the understanding of my three beautiful children.

Thanks to Matthew and Scott for your photos in this book. Words cannot express my appreciation for Pastor Tony and Trish Jackson, LaToya Taite—Headspeth, Sherika, my beautiful cousin, and Denise Thibeault, who all assisted me in this publication. To all of the natural hair models that worked on this and other projects that have shown the world that natural is beautiful. They have clearly shown we must embrace the natural within.

A special acknowledgement goes to my inspirational confident Dr. Sirretta Williams, mother of Laveranues Cole, television host, public figure, author, business owner, and city and community activist in Jacksonville, FL.

I also want to thank all my friends and prayer partners for you love and inspiration on this project.Thank you Mrs. Marsena Cook for the final edit and Ashley Thomas the content review and assistance in this publication.

PREFACE

As a graduate of Bethune-Cookman College (BCC) in 1996, I understand that research, knowledge, and exchange are great valuable aspects of my professional development. Almost 60 years ago, Dr. Mary McLeod Bethune left her legacy that influenced everyone that touched the campus of Bethune-Cookman College. Her passion for research influenced me to dig deeper into understanding how chemicals we use daily affect our health. Mary McLeod Bethune was not only an educator, but she was also a leader, community activist, an explorer, and innovator. She was an inspiration to so many individuals, inventors, and business owners. Working side by side with her former student and friend Marjorie Joyner, they formed the United Beauty Organization, an organization that focused on quality hair care. Their efforts lead to the advancement in the hair care industry today. Marjorie Joyner was not just an average student when she stepped into Bethune-Cookman College. She was already well known for her passion for hair care. She invented a permanent wave machine, in 1928, which became a permanent possession of her former boss Madame CJ Walker (formerly Sarah Breedlove). It is just ironic that former slaves developed the platform of what our hair care industry is today. After Marjorie completed her cosmetology education at Bethune-Cookman College, she became the National Advisor and advocate for over 200 students of Madame Walkers Beauty School. Exploring history helps us understand the origin of our hair care, and beauty secrets that impact our future.

Working in the medical field for over 20 years, I have witnessed the devastating effects of diseases. I often find that my opportunity to educate people about preventative measures is missed. This is why I share this passion and I believe that if science, medicine, and the hair care industry come together we can create an amazing platform for our world.
I am a health care professional, and I currently travel globally as a natural hair consultant. I began an initiative to help others understand the health benefits to going natural, and also to help others understand alternatives to hair care. Please feel free to contact me at orjanette@ yahoo.com for your personalized hair care plan. I am available to give you researched guidance to help improve your hair care. **Nubia's Guide for Natural Hair Care** is a global reference guide to give you the fundamental secrets to hair care.

FOREWORD

This book is dedicated to all the Queens and Kings who once allowed the chemicals to strip you from your fundamental beauty.

Embrace the person you see in the mirror, your hair does not define your beauty.

DISCLAIMER

This book contains my personal experiences, some research, tips from v-loggers, and safe alternatives to hair care. I am not a beautician and I do not discourage the use of your styling professional.

TRANSITION

Questions you must ask yourself prior to transitioning to natural.

1. Have you lost your hair around the edges or is your hair thinning?
2. Do you suffer from migraines or mental confusions?
3. Do you have severe heavy menstrual cramping, problems with your cycle, or bleeding?
4. Is your hair healthy?
5. Do you require oil in your hair daily to keep your hair shine and to reduce breakage?
6. Are you noticing more shedding when you comb or brush your hair?
7. Have you found a good shampoo?
8. Are you suffering from medical problems like Diabetes, HTN, Thyroid problems, or Cancer?
9. Is there a strong family history of Dementia?

HAIR FACT

The hair is mainly protein with cuticles that overlap. Hair grows about 1 cm – ½ inches each month. Women ages 16-24 years old typically have the most hair growth, and men normally grow hair faster than women. Between the ages of 40-50 hair becomes dry and you will notice 20% of the hair is lost. Proper diet and a good health status will improve your hair growth. Oils are produced from your own sebum, which helps protect and seal your hair from damage. Cutting back on caffeine or other stimulants helps improve your hair and increases the circulation to the scalp, which aids in hair growth. Hormones, poor handling, and poor diet may contribute to hair loss. An increase of water helps your hair grow in addition to biotin supplements.

Before you begin your natural hair journey, you should determine the reason why you should go natural. Natural is only a transition from the old processed look to a more natural, appearance. Transitioning from the chemically relaxed hair to natural is one of the healthiest choices anyone could ever make. Cutting your old hair is not always an easy transition but as a health care professional and consultant it is my role to help you understand the vital importance of going natural. There are multiple health benefits when you go natural, and when most people wear their hair natural they become more conscious of their innate beauty. If you have young daughters or granddaughters, look at them. I hope you can see beauty in a different way. We need to explore and understand true value of beauty. Your hair has little to do with the image we portray according to the European culture. People from other countries of the world are baffled at the Afro-American hiding their God given natural beauty. Big hair is attractive and well worth the embracement. People of different cultures and nationalities admire the big hair. We all have to learn how to embrace our hair as well, whether you are African American or not.

Some important facts about going natural are worth exploration. Transitioning to natural hair can save you money, stimulate hair growth, help you become healthier, and you can get very creative by exploring some beautiful, unique styles with little to no effort. People face their fears about wearing tight coils, kinky hair, and/or nappy hair. Understand the word nappy is not necessarily negative. According to the Urban Dictionary, "It is simply tightly coiled and unaltered curled hair." I share some of my personal experiences and why I have transformed my nappy to happy. I hope to make your natural hair journey a smooth transition.

Chemically relaxing of the hair destroys your hair by changing the pH. Your normal hair pH is low with a more complex range – more acid ranging from 3—to about 5 pH. Chemical relaxer has a high pH ranging about 10-13 on the scale, and it breaks open the cortex and destroys the bonds of your hair. Chemicals change the molecular structure of the hair follicle, along with destroying and weakening your hair. The combination of oil and water are important for healthy hair. Because oil and water are not soluble, they are equally required to penetrate the hair follicle. This combination is needed to seal and protect the cuticle for all types of hair. When your hair is chemically relaxed it loses its natural ability to produce oils and your hair becomes compromised due to dullness, dryness, and breakage.

Although natural hair may appear dull and lack luster, the hair is normally enriched with it's own sebum or oil from the cuticles. Natural, unprocessed hair is much healthier. The ends of the natural hair require a bit more focus when you are styling your hair, because less oil is noted the further you get from the cortex of the hair. Sebaceous glands are found deep into the scalp near the outer root sheath of the hair. If you don't properly protect and care for the ends of your hair it can result in splitting, dead ends, and breakage.

Less oil is necessary when you are going natural because your body regularly produces its own oil. Hormones affect your hair growth. I recommend good nutrition and hydration. Chemically relaxed, damaged, and traumatized hair is stripped from the natural ability to stretch, protect and seal. Chemicals affect your internal oil glands and make your hair very dry, dull, and less shiny. The severity of the chemical destruction varies from person to person, but (trust me) the more chemicals applied, the more you are at risk for damage. Damaged hair and traumatized hair requires Emergency 911 treatment. Deep conditioning and pH stabilizer are required to prevent future hair loss or damage. Find a skilled hair professional that will be honest and help you set realistic goals for your hair. Hair trauma requires the help from a trained salon professional to reduce further damage. When you seek help, you must be willing to seek a corrective action plan to get your hair back in shape. Your stylist needs to know your medical problems, medication, standard styling techniques, stress, products you are using, and what your personal goals are for your hair. Don't be surprised if the stylist tells you there is nothing they can do to help you especially if you have hereditary alopecia. Sounds awful, but the truth is some people are predestined to hair loss. Unfortunately, hormones play a significant role in hair loss, but a hair restoration specialist will guide you further on the alopecia and assist you with finding a good conditioning treatment and encourage stopping all chemicals. Finding a salon that focuses on healthy hair rehab is a big challenge. My goal is to encourage salons to tap into hair restorative care, by educating them about the products and harmful effects so they can teach their clients how to focus on healthy hair care. Good nutrition, hydration, and exercise help speed the recovery during the rehabilitation of your hair. See my care plan to assist in your hair care needs.

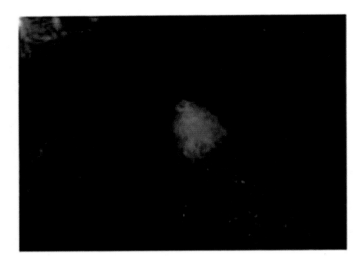

Creamy crack addiction requires rehab. This rehab starts from the inside out. Salons need to help people avoid the addictions and provide therapeutic options for their clients. I've heard women say they will stop perming their hair temporary until their hair grows back. Returning to the old ways of applying the creamy crack, the perms, the dyes, and the other junk is contraindicated when you are going natural. Going natural requires healthier habits. Become more interconnected with the beautiful person you are without the cosmetic or chemical dependencies.

Coloring or dyeing the hair also destroys the hair. After coloring your hair the damage begins. You will notice lots of shedding and your hair loses its natural ability to produce sebum and repair itself. After coloring the hair don't be surprised by the fact it may take up to six months to grow back a healthy hair.

Stop asking your friends, with a thick lustrous head of hair about their secret to their mane. Your friends should tell you to stop chemically processing, relaxing, and coloring your hair to see a better emotional, mental, and physical balance. Over the last few years, we have become much smarter about the perms, but we can't negate the fact that hair coloring is much worse. Women are perming four times a year, which is a big improvement from relaxing the hair every six weeks. Letting go of the chemical relaxer is very difficult, especially if you love the silky feel of your freshly relaxed hair. For several reasons, I just don't miss chemically relaxing my hair; for example, the burning of the scalp causes ridiculous sores in my scalp. The sores and lesions you get from burning your scalp exemplify the unreasonable old saying, "No pain no gain." Those nasty lesions pre-exposed you to cancer. Anything that breaks down the natural mucous or your genetic makeup can cause cancer. Manmade chemicals cause cancer. Think about this: people love spicy foods, but the spice causes ulcers. Your body triggers or sends signals to the brain that say this is not good for you, but you eat the spicy food and then you suffer the most excruciating pain. People just love pain! You try to find an antacid to stop the burning effect. Once the burning occurs there is no Band-Aid to cover the damage. Ulcers are precancerous lesions, just like scalp burns potentiate cancer.

Let's explore the damage from the dyes. It is all pretty scary! Dye damage causes death. Dyes destroy the protein and moisture balance of the hair. Peroxide is strong, and it lifts the cuticles. People with curly, short hair notice a great effect from coloring the hair. Please be aware severe allergic reactions are a potential from the use of dyes. I would never advise hair coloring to someone wearing their hair long. Typically people with low porous hair experience good results from hair dye for cosmetic appearances and their hair feels much harder from the use of the coloring, but please do not color your hair if you want a long mane because any alteration to your normal molecular structure of your hair may cause more breakage. Sometimes the cuticles are so tight that water and oil doesn't enter into the hair shaft. Typically the hair is strong, with a nice curl pattern, and appears very soft. But hair porosity is more of a challenge for salons, because salons generalize the hair care from person to person based on the appearance of the hair (see the section of this book that explains how to test your hair for porosity to understand the importance of testing and the best hair care solutions for porous problems). Styling is much easier for people with low porous hair, who dye their hair. Dyed hair becomes more flexible, and the hair accepts the protein and conditioners; typically protein is added to most styling products. Not to get too deep into why dying hair can be beneficial, at this time I will have to explore it in another book at another time. There is just a lot for you to know about hair, and you will never get all the information in one place. But my research helps us understand more about the hair, and I challenge you to do your own research. Read all product labels before using any product and understand your hair care needs.

Going natural is not an easy transition for everyone. Some women struggle with the "Big Chop." The big chop is when you cut all chemically process hair and transition your hair back to its natural state (or go back to a virgin like appearance.) Transitioning is not an easy process. So many women fear the unknown. They imagine themselves going from the European straight, long hair to the natural, shrunken Afro. To help you visualize the image you can put your ponytail in a tight bun and make sure your hair is up this gives you the best appearance of what you will look like with short hair. As you look into the mirror, you will to envision yourself in a whole new way. When women do the big chop, it may be necessary to wear makeup and accessorize a little more to have a real appreciation for the new look. The biggest surprise after the big chop is not always the length but the texture. Hair texture is so unpredictable; you can't assume your hair texture is the same as your mother and siblings. Study your hair to help determine your hair care needs, know your hair type for the best guidance and styling tips shared from your favorite internet vlogger will improve your appearance. Hair typing is not a definitive guide, but it helps you understand more about products that may work best for you. After you become more comfortable with your hair type and your hair's porosity, you will understand your hair requirements are different. Honestly, the best transition comes from the shaving of the head completely to the scalp. The boy cut is easy to work with, and you don't have to worry about cutting the ends for a while because there are no splitting or damage. Plus once you cut the hair to one length you should notice growth at an even rate. Think about how seeds grow, they form into a plant if the root is kept watered and the weather conditions are favorable. Plant grows into a tree just like your hair grows. Start nourishing from the root and you will yield a good crop. As you transition from a boy cut, shaved hair almost to the scalp you will have a better idea of hair growth. During each phase of growth of your hair you will learn vital information about hair care needs.

Go back to the basics! Keep it simple and cover the scalp when the weather conditions change. Growth from the shortest cut is extreme, but your transition journey will become more exciting as you watch your hair grow. Most ladies who transition notice a vast amount of growth during the first year to 18 months. Keeping the hair moisturized and hydrated makes the hair grow more. Take note the ends of the hair appear much healthier when you cut your hair to the scalp. Your hair requires less product if you do the big chop. Keep your scalp healthy and watch yourself transition to a healthier you.

Take photos during each stage of your transition so that you can measure the progressions of your transformation. Photos help empower you and help you embrace your new look.

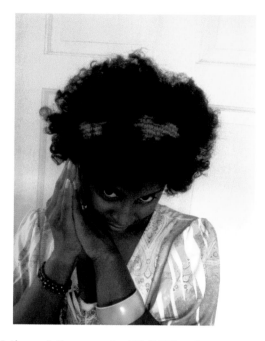

Mirror, Mirror on the Wall Who do you see...

Like the witch from Snow White, look into the mirror, and tell me who do you see?

I was scared to look at the hair that was curled up so tight, like that little fro from below.

I see the man minus the WOW!

I see the coward who was afraid to accept her flaws.

I see a woman who was lost, trapped, and held captive to into this delusional fairy tale.

I see something missing looking at me.

I don't even know this person who is looking at me.

I see a challenge in the path that lies before me.

I see a woman who wanted so much to be like the other woman, full of envy, and jealousy.

I see the perplexed individual looking at me;

Words can't seem to define the natural beauty looking in the mirror.

This transformation is deep and only the Mirror can help you understand how going natural change my world!

This poem is an expression of the mixed emotions we have when we first transition to natural. People feel confused and lost. Comments are made but the public has no idea what is really going on in your head when you first transition. It saddens me to know that the validation of our beauty has been a misconception we held on to for centuries. Struggling with your real birth-given beauty and society trends or normalcy is why so many women hide behind the mask to conceal their true beauty. The big chop and short hair does not reflect the beauty I thought I once had when I wore the wigs. The first glimpse of yourself may be a shock because you may remind yourself of your father, brother, or even some relative, the fact that you are still a woman. Try to accentuate your new look with a little eye makeup, some big earrings, bright colors, and maybe a headpiece. Make sure you look into the mirror again and take some photos to see how you will shift and develop into the true person you are today. Be bold, be proud, and love the beautiful woman that radiates strength, character, and charm.

There are so many different grades of hair which makes hair typing very confusing. To simplify, the hair typing guide I created a simple guide to help you understand hair typing. There are four categories. The traditional hair typing scale ranges from 1A to the 4 C hair type.

- Hair type one (1) is bone straight, the hair of an Asian. This hair is straight.
- Hair Type two (2) can be a Caucasian person that has straight hair. You may see some curve shape to the hair.
- Hair Type three (3) is very similar to your mixed race, or the Hispanics who typically have more elongated curl pattern or the curl is a more definitive S Shape.
- Hair type four (4) is common for African Americans. African American hair type is not limited to a 4c to a 5-type hair it can go also into the type 2 or 3 hair type. Because there are so many variations of African American hair the hair typing scale may be limited. My hair type guide may be very limited because the new hair typing categorizations has expanded from 1 to 5 hair types. The letters represent the curl or coil pattern, and it can range from a slight wave A to an F, which is tight, springy hair that does not move, and maintains its shape and style.
- A – Is classified as fine or thin hair.
- B – Is classified as Medium hair.
- C – Is classified as coarse hair.

You may also find safe hair care products in your kitchen to treat dandruff, nourish, cleanse, and help improve the overall appearance of your hair. Edible products are relatively safe for your hair. Your hair is a living cell and hair food works great to keep the living cells from dying; therefore, most edible products like eggs are an excellent source of protein for the hair. All living cells require water, oxygen, and food to grow healthy and strong.

It was thought that the Nessler's use of cow urine and water in 1896. It was the first process that changed the chemical structure of the hair, according to some sources. We do know that perms alter the hairs pH. Perms are all caustic because they burn and destroy. Remember perms used by Caucasians gives them curls, but the Afro-American perm smoothes out the curls and straightens the hair. Upon review of the history, I concluded we are a very complicated when it comes to our hair. Smoothing out the edges to straighten the kinks was not the original intent of the perm. With a hair-rolling technique, the use of the chemicals creates curly hair. Hair care comes in so many different options, and I think we have lost our focus on accepting ourselves.

Garrett Augustus Morgan, a child of a formal slave from Kentucky, accidently discovered the first hair relaxer for African Americans. He worked in a factory in which he revealed that the chemicals he used to repair a sewing machine somehow relaxed curly hair and made it straight. He tested his chemical on an Airedale dog, a dog that has a curly coat of hair — and found that the chemical made the dog's hair straight. Poor dog, tormented by the application of the alkaline chemical to his fur; today he would be charged with animal cruelty. In 1913 G.A. Morgan went on to expand his business to straighten or relax the hair. His company is known as G.A. Morgan Hair Refining Company. He also had other inventions that are very prominent to African Americans.

In 1890, Madame CJ Walker worked in a laundry house, and she suffered from alopecia from a scalp disorder. She became the first to produce the scalp conditioning and healing formula. Her growth serums and hair care products are rich with Sulfur to enhance the growth of the hair. She became the first millionaire to invite us to the hair care solution from the South. Madame CJ was the daughter of a slave, and she married at a very early age. Madame CJ Walker was also known as Sarah Breedlove prior to her marriage. She is the originator of our hair care and beauty industry for African Americans. Her product campaign read, "have a reason to envy another girl, her lovely hair, and her charming complication." I find this advertisement concerning because it became a misconception of our true heritage, skin lightening, hair straighten, and more. Madame CJ Walker's hair care products promote lots of growth because they contained a powerful antibacterial agent known as Sulfur. In 1910, she traveled to Kentucky in search of finding a home or factory, to continue to expand on her products and her hair care, super growing hair care, and conditioning treatment. It's an interesting fact that she went to the hometown of the inventor of the perm, Garrett Morgan — to expand sales on her product and services. These prominent businesswomen influenced Garrett Morgan, and he launched his company three years later in 1913. The first perm was an extremely harsh alkaline product that caused the destruction of the bonds of the hair and also caused the hair's normal pH 3-5 to change the pH to 10-13. Garrett Morgan needed to find a way to reduce the damage from the relaxer. Madame CJ Walker had a solution to growing hair. She made millions through her success to the hair industry.

In 1905 Madame Walker invented a conditioning treatment for straightening hair. In 1945 Marjorie Joyner, graduated from Bethune Cookman College. She worked side by side with Mary McLeod Bethune to keep the legacy of Madame Walker to improve the hair care industry for all African Americans. Today our hair care industry is what it is because of their contributions. Madame CJ Walker employed Marjorie whom invented the permanent wave machine, which straightened black hair and added extended curls to Caucasian hair, but she never received a patent to her invention. It became the property of Madam CJ Walker's Company. Through Madame Walker and Marjorie's friendship they started the funding for the United Beauty School, which focused on the development and the quality of hair care for African Americans.

Black women finally understand how to embrace the kinks. I noticed more Caucasian's attraction to wearing my big Afro and embracing my kinks. What is the fascination with the Afro puff? The hair looks like cotton and for some reason, the master was not interested in picking the cotton back in the day, and now he can't keep his hands out of the Afro hair. The "Do not touch my natural hair campaign" is a campaign to help people understand that touching of a natural women's hair is like a violation to her core. I witness a white man touching the Afro puff, and he said he wondered what he could do to get his hair like a little girl's hair. Watching the response of the little girl and a grandmother, the little girl avoided responding, but the look on the grandmother's face said it all. It seems like she wanted to hit him across the face. He was a minister, so she resisted the temptation to react, but that look said what gives you the right to touch her hair. It was almost like he had just grabbed her butt and she wanted to slap the heaven out of him. I can't understand why men of different ethnicities are so fascinated with the feel and touch of the natural hair. Touching natural hair creates frizz and destroys the styling. Please don't touch the hair! A women's hair signifies her ethnical power. Similar to the power Samson lost from the cutting of his hair.

CONFESSIONS OF THE CREAMY CRACK ADDICT

Creamy crack addiction is simply jargon naturalistas use to describe their addiction to the creamy hair relaxers. During my experience with the chemical relaxer: I was in quest for something that provided my hair with a silky soft feeling. I needed something that made me feel like an African queen. I had this false sense that chemicals and products even without the relaxer were going to satisfy my quench for those nasty affects like I had from the relaxers. I just did not know I was so addicted to the stuff. When I first went natural, I must have had over 500 dollars worth of product in my bathroom. Products like the perm just are not enough for you! Products may not burn as a relaxer, but it sure is addictive. I just wanted some more junk to change the feel of my natural hair. Chemical addiction is a real problem, and it requires therapy. If you don't believe me just watch all the effects from all the chemicals. Creamy crack burns, causes cancer, gives head sores, and even causes memory loss.

The cost of the creamy crack or hair relaxers dropped significantly to markdown low. The creamy crack distribution companies needed to reinvent another way to make a profit. I tried to warn the salons that natural clients wanted more services that met their needs. So many women became tired of the harmful effects of the chemicals, so they just stopped perming or chemically straightening their hair. They started wearing hair weave in which cost around $250-$500 for the hairpieces alone. On June 7, 2012 I posted on Facebook a sale of $.99 cents for the African Pride hair relaxer. I received a ton of response to the "get your creamy crack stockpile while supplies last". What on earth are we doing to our hair? I should have posted "get your cancer causing chemicals while supplies last". I don't know if perms will become obsolete like the cigarettes, but they are working its way off the shelves.

Everyone loves the silk like, fresh feeling of the relaxed hair! I personally just don't miss the perm for several reasons. For example, the burning of the scalp was ridiculous and I dreaded the sores created on my scalp from the harsh chemicals. The lesions acquired from the chemical burns to your scalp are only a false reassurance of the old saying, "No pain, no gain." The pain theory is bogus because the little nasty lesions pre-exposed you to cancer. Remember anything that breaks the natural mucosa or your genetic makeup can potentiate cancer. This is a sad reality, but manmade materials used improperly cause cancers. Think about this, you love spicy foods, but spicy foods can cause ulcers. Your body sends signals to the brain to say this is not good for you, but you eat the spicy foods and then you suffer from the most excruciating pain. People just love pain! You try to find an antacid to stop the burn, but unfortunately the burning effect continues because the irritation or sore are created and there is no Band-Aid to cover the damage. Ulcers are precancerous just like scalp trauma may trigger cancer cells.

You ever saw someone beating themselves in the head? They claim they beat to prevent them from scratching their scalp before the perming process. Some creamy crack addicts say the constant itching of the scalp is an indication that their hair needs relaxing. This misconception is truly creamy crack addictions at its best!

I say go see your doctor and get some Ativan. Please don't get offended about the term 'creamy crack'; it is simply jargon we use for any addiction to stuff that just is not good for you. Creamy crack makes you beat your head in public; it really looks like you need to be locked up in the psych ward. I honestly can't say anything good about the creamy crack causing burning or scalp lesions. I have even heard creamy crack addicts say, "If I don't use the relaxers to my hair will fall out". Get real people! Going through such extreme measures to get that hair straight like the sores, the burning, and the disease caused by chemicals just is not worth the pain to me anymore. Chemical burning is no lye, perming of the hair or the addiction to any chemical is just not good! Let me explain the true feeling you get when you apply the chemical relaxer to the scalp. It feels like acid being poured on the scalp. I am sure you could image the tears, pain, and unimaginable desire to throw my head in the toilet as the intense heat radiated from my scalp to my brain. Whoever said 'no pain no gain' need to be ashamed of themselves, because anything that causes that much pain is not worth it to me anymore.

Creamy crack addicts invest significant money in their hair care. They went into the salon, and came out looking the same way they looked when they went into the salon. I have to say I never felt any significant difference when I went into the salon than I did after I came out of the salon. I just wanted some magic for my hair. My hair was the same going into the salon as it was before I went in; my hair would appear temporarily luscious. Creamy crack addicts invest lots of money on products, salons services and wigs, because of their own lack the self worth. I admit this has been a challenge for me also I even thought at one time if I colored my hair blonde it would enhance the beauty of my dark chocolate skin.

I remember leaving my thick head of hair at the salon. I keep feeling my hair and thinking to myself what the blank happened to my hair, my head was full of sores. I even remember the stylist telling me just to apply some Neosporin to my irritated scalp. Yes, I just paid 100 dollars for a bunch of sores in my scalp from the chemicals, and then was told to go home and apply some Neosporin! I think once you've experienced hair trauma you should evaluate the junk applied to your head. There are damaging effects of the creamy crack and you must be careful. Once the perms begin to burn there is no easy solution to washing it out. Too much washing can cause hair loss.

When I became natural, I still had a real problem; I would try anything and everything because I wanted to control my curls or the frizz. The frizz was out of control, untamed curls, or tufts.

I just needed some creamy crack to fix the problem. I would layer my hair with product, so heavy my hair felt like it had weights holding it down. I used some of the thickest creamiest curl taming solutions there was on the market, until my daughter said, "Mommy, please wash your hair because the flakes, and product sitting on your hair look nasty." I realized my creamy crack addiction to perms and lye turned into creamy crack addiction to styling products. I don't want to be insulting anyone's products, but every product on the market is not for everyone. I thought that if I layer enough products my hair would look just like the girl on the advertisement material. I purchased all kinds of creams, gels, and other hair care products until I realized I went way over the budget again. I was spending more money on products than I would have if I had just gone to the salon. I felt like a product junkie and realized I needed help! Be aware of the creamy crack addiction; it is just not the best solution for growth or a head of healthy hair. I advise you who are addicted to the creamy crack to go to an education hair expo and learn more about the things we can do to our hair that will help it grow and look healthier.

I am amazed when my little 10-year-old girl (who has at least 10-12 inches of hair) told me "Please Mommy, don't straighten my hair". She loves her curls and embraces her natural look. She reminds me regularly it is not important to her to show the length of her hair.

She embraces the time we share as I manage her mane. Because her mane is very thick more detangling and preparation is necessary; she doesn't mind sitting for over two hours because she is always satisfied with the outcome. I also embrace the mommy and daughter time we spend when I do her hair. Giving your daughter the confidence and helping her understand her beauty. Braiding or other styling is a valuable time created from mothers as they style their daughter's hair. Help your babies love their own hair and understand their beauty. Break generational curses by giving your daughter a sense of her real sense of worth. I want us all to help our children to understand the importance of leaving the slave mentality in the past. We are free, and it is acceptable just to be yourself. Wear your hair any way you like, but be careful about the spirit of seduction. You may even experience curl envy and begin to hate your own hair because you want your hair to reach the standards of someone else. Big hair, long hair, silky, straight hair can be very seductive to others, and there may be a spirit of jealousy. Be aware of the curse that was passed on from generation to generation. We are all different. We must learn to embrace ourselves, and never create a false sense of worth based on someone else's standards.

FITTING NATURAL HAIR CARE INTO YOUR BUDGET

Since the economy changes in 2008, rise in fuel, food, and cost of living women have become wiser. Instead of paying that $200—$400 to the salon for styles that was never intended for you we begin styling our hair on a budget. Women faced the reality of paying their rent or getting their hair done. If this is your reality you may want to regroup and evaluate some things. Extra expenditures that are not in the budget like getting your hair styling versus paying the baby sitter are just something unimaginable. People say to me, "Why you don't pamper yourself?" I explain because my hair care does not take precedence over my responsibilities. Imagine walking around looking like everything was in order in your life, you are looking like a Ford model; your hair is perfect, when in all reality you need some more money to put food in the refrigerator. This is a mental bondage! There are ways to get your hair done, and not break your budget. I always sought options to hair care when I felt it was necessary. At an early age I began working with my own hair, and I had someone very special that always guide me through the path of making it look correct. Trust me sometimes it was not too pretty! My friends would tell me to fix the look, but to tell the truth we all were in a learning phase back then and no one really knew what to do with their hair. Self-help video guides are now available to improve your styling dilemmas. Women can look nice even on a tight budget.

Hairstyles should not be expensive and should fit into your budget. When you create a budget, you should include your hair care expenditures or your salon expensive. We want the world to see us as though we have no concerns at all, when in reality we have masked the fact that we had to borrow money to get our hair done. The untouchable look creates a false sense of security and others will avoid any interference with the shell created around you. Learning to live on a budget and finding alternative ways to achieve a nice look are easily obtainable. Having a new natural way of thinking, loving, and embracing the real you and managing your budget will have a profound impact on your confidence. Others around you will see the real person. I am not suggesting people should go around untidy and unkempt. I am simply suggesting you embrace yourself. You can include your hair care on a budget. Believe me even on a budget you can find different option for alternate occasions. When you step into a corporate setting, wedding, or any big event, no one will ever know that you are on a budget.

Make it blonde, straight, and long! Hair coloring is another expenditure we never put into our budget. Ladies I challenge you to be conscious about the cost of your hair care. Women are learning how to weave and create lace wigs for their hair, and have found that it promotes a healthy financial balance. Going natural can be just as costly as going to the salon. Products can destroy a budget if you are in quest for the ultimate styling aid or growth serum. Your average product junkie is not afraid to pay the maximum amount for products whether they are effective or not. When I first went natural, I was searching for the ultimate growing serum. I invested much in Miss Jessie's products (loved her Christmas deals). I loved Carol's Daughter, until I had the hardest time finding her products and I even trying to become a distributor. I learned the hair care products did not make my hair grow and styling creams wore my hair down, which creates a heavy feeling. All the products I used required lots of clarifying shampoo, which only stripped my hair of its own natural oils. After I studied and realized my best options was to keep it simple. I use more natural oils like coconut oil, jojoba, almond and olive oil. Oils that can be ingested or edible are relatively safe for your mane. Coconut oil lasts for days and allows an excellent balance for most hair types including those who have low porous hair.

Low porous hair doesn't sink to the bottom when immersed in water. This type hair dries fast and most people don't have to worry about nasty scalp infections created by fungus, yeast, or mold. Flaking of the scalp may not be a problem with the low porous hair, but product flaking may be prominent due to lack of absorption. Low porous hair doesn't care for too many products either. After about 2 days the low porous hair will require washing to remove all the flake and product build up. Low porous hair does not allow water to penetrate into the hair follicle, due to tight bonding of the cuticles. PH stabilizers and humectants work well for low porous hair. Glycerin really helps with products, water, and oil for more absorption. Humectants help with hydration. Glycerin is great humectants because it draws moisture from the atmosphere. Moisture is needed to increase hydration balance to your hair. Glycerin allows low porous hair to hold on to the water molecules longer, therefore creating more absorption with the oils. Remember if you use products clarification will be needed to cleanse the hair within 3 days, or you might be looking like you have lice.

Be aware of product shopping; it is not a good habit. You might want to avoid being the first to try or test the products on the shelf. Without adequate usage of any product you will never know the full potential of the products. If you don't know your hair I recommend you test your new products for about 3 weeks before switching to something different. It may not hurt to try new products, but remember to stay within your budget. I highly recommend you stay on your worry-free hair care regimen and determine what works best for you, without adding new products to your hair care regimen. Too many products used at the same time can cause a buildup. Products you hold on to for any length of time may not be beneficial due to the alterations in its potency. Simply get rid of the outdated product. As a mixologist, I caution you that all products have an expiration date. I love combining my own growth serums containing flax seed, coconut oil, aloe Vera, tree tea, grape seed oil, and jojoba oil; but I noticed after 30 days the serum began to lose its full benefit and began to spoil. I assumed the antibacterial properties of the tree tea oil would prevent it from spoiling, but Aloe Vera turns brown if it is not refrigerated and kept in a dark, cool place.

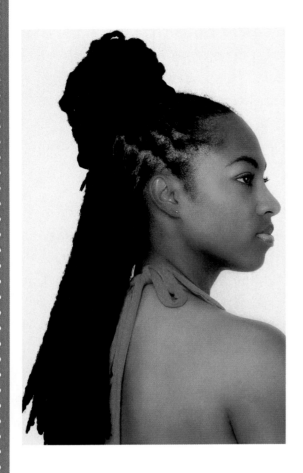

If you want to know what products works best for your hair, I recommend you go to YouTube select a vlogger that has similar hair to your hair type; and then check out Curlmart to match your hair type with the products that is recommended specifically for you.

NUBIA'S SIMPLE STEPS TO GROWTH

Most women go natural for hair growth. To grow hair successful, you must know the fundamentals of hair care. Exploring with different chemicals may cause fluctuations in your hair growth. Chemical straightening of your hair causes breakage, and there is no definitive solution to hair growth. Chemical relaxing and processing causes thinning of your hair, and trust me, over time the damage may be irreversible and cause permanent hair loss. Chemical relaxers contain lye or no lye. Perms alter the pH balance of the hair, and our hair transform from a natural acidic state to an alkaline state. You can try so many products to help correct the pH imbalance of the hair after perming it, but the truth is that the traumatic alteration is damaging and it effects your hair growth. Natural virgin hair is healthy with a low pH (ranging from a 3-5.5 range) the strands may or may not be tightly bonded, textures are different, and hair type can be categorized from 1a to 5f. 1 hair type is hair that has no wave pattern, and the hair is bone straight; typical people of Asian culture have this hair type. The 4 or 5 hair types are Afro-centric hair, and it has lots of kinks, coils, and knots, which is how you determine the lettering of the hair by the curl pattern. Curl pattern and definition determine the lettering of your hair. Typically Afro-American hair may or may not have a definite curl, and it may be very difficult to determine the true hair type. Coarse hair is the best way to describe the 4-5-type hair. Coarse hair requires a little more work to style, but the advantage is that no hair spray is required to keep the hair in place.

Hair typing scale is very debatable with all the variations of hair. Most people use it as a guide to help them determine the best hair care options. Consider the traditional scale stopped at 4E, but don't be surprised to see the hair typing scale extended. Hair typing is only a guide to help us understand hair similarities. Hair growth should be realistic, and you should never compare your hair type growth to others that come from different cultures. Learn what works best for you. Personally I like the wash n go because it works without the applications of thick products for my 4 C hair. Some literature recommends creamy products for the styling of the 4 c hair to help weigh the hair down to make the curl appear elongated or stretched. My hair has the pH problem and products cake up. For my hair growth, it is easier to keep my hair clean and not focus too much on the styling aids. If you know anything about hair that pulls and pops, you'll understand my rationale on why less works best for some of us. Some hair requires pH—balanced products. You can test your product with a Litmus test strip to determine if your products are more acidic versus alkaline. If the product is acidic the pH is low at 3.5-5.5, the products may work better, but be forewarned a low pH may cause breakage to the hair also. Try some vinegar for a clarifying cleansing. Remember your grandmother telling you to use vinegar after you over processed your hair from the perm to help reverse the damage? It napped your hair right up, but remember once the damage has destroyed the hair it will fall out. Try to dilute vinegar to improve your ph balance. Baking soda is also another great cleaner because it brings your hair to a neutral balance. Baking soda is cheap and one of the best clarifier. I don't recommend mixing the baking soda and the vinegar although you will find so many hair vloggers demonstrating that. Chemicals strip your hair! Again time, patience, and the constant reevaluation of your knowledge of your hair care needs will improve your outcome.

Hair is unique and should be treated differently depending on the circumstances. Stress, medical conditions, poor handling, and weather changes alter hair growth. Do you desire bigger hair? Stop stressing, comb less, keep the hair clean, nourish it, and watch it grow. See the sections later in the book to determine how to improve your growth and deal with issues with natural hair.

Although weaved hair is a protective styling, you can damage your hair from the pulling too tight. Tight pulling causes tension. Any poor scalp care or tension can create as much damage as any chemicals , so therefore weaves can be more damaging and that is no lye. Hair needs air and the scalp needs a little sun, water, and minerals from the environment. Most people want to know how to achieve the long mane. For different reasons, people go natural. I began noticing my edges were thinning, and everyone in my family has thin edges. I was determined not to let it happen to me, so I stopped using chemical straightening of my hair for nine months. I loved the versatility of the different styles and wearing hair weaves. I became disgusted with my hair, and I did my big chop without planning it. It was the day before my pop's funeral, two days before Christmas 2007. I had no idea what I was doing, and I did not even care at that moment. Everyone was too distraught, and no one had much to say not even about my new nappy hair. No one acknowledged how nice my fro looked! I guess my radical and random behaviors were not uncommon to my family; they love me no matter what.

Now I understand your big chop does not determine hair growth. Growth depends on multiple factors. I studied to determine what makes my hair grow. I wonder if hair growth is determined by the use of vitamins, genes, or is it lack of manipulations. There is no definitive answer to hair growth, but we all grow hair each month, some people retain their length, and don't shed as much.

Exercise and scalp massages are great options for stimulating hair grow. To clarify the myth that cutting your hair makes your hair grow faster, you need to know your hair will grow every six weeks whether you cut your hair or not. Cutting your hair does not accelerate growth. Clipping the dead ends is important because the ends require a good moisture balance. Don't forget the hydration is the key to health strong hair. Handling and manipulating our hair is critical. If you have a hard time detangling your hair, you will create more split ends break and destroy your cuticles. Hair porosity can also cause damage. Be aware that some products complicate the porosity, tangling process so know your products, and understand how they work.

Your scalp should always be clean. Keep your pores free of thick sealants that trap dirt, bacteria, and other debris. Homeopathic secrets can help reduce shedding. There are things that you can try at home that are not prescribed by a doctor, such as the use of caffeine rinses to enhance the conditioning process. Some people use tea bags and coffee rinses prior to the deep conditioners to help stimulate the scalp. Believe it or not, salt helps with hydration. Haven't you ever heard the old saying that dirty hair is healthy? Well, that's true because dirt has salt bonds and other minerals that help the hair with a moisture balance. The use of clay helps detoxify my scalp, and the clay also adds minerals to help improve growth. Clays like Rhassoul and Bentonite clay are great for people are suffering from diseases or have anemia. There are some great detoxification methods you can use like clay. Heavy metals like aluminum, lead, mercury, chemicals and minerals deposited in the hair cause lots of breakage. These elements need to be removed without striping your hair through a clarification process. Our hair requires a good balance of sodium, potassium, and calcium in order to remain viable. I would recommend the use of detoxification only on a monthly or maybe even every 6 months. Bentonite clay, Moroccan red clay, Rhassoul clay, and Aztec clay have been used for centuries. The clay allows the ion and the metals from the earth to assist with mineral replacement that is necessary for growth. This is a great option for the salon willing to provide you this service because it is relaxing and beneficial in so many ways. I love detoxification with any of the clays because it really helps add and remove important elements for people with anemia or anyone who may have just completed cancer treatment. Detoxification is a great way to help your body recover from the minerals missing, to promote healthy hair after any medical crisis, and correcting issues from head to toe will promote healthy cells.

There are multiple things you can do to help hair like pre-poo, no combing, regularly detangling with a Denman brush and use of organic products or pure oils. See a beautician or dermatologist if you don't notice any growth or if you are experiencing scalp problems. Protective styling is excellent for the reduction of shedding. A satin bonnet works well to keep the hair protected from the UV rays and climate changes.

Scalp massages are very beneficial. Scalp stimulation improves the blood flow to the scalp. Your scalp doesn't get enough stimulation. I highly recommend you could go to the salon weekly to get the deep stimulation treatment and be placed a corrective action plan to make your hair grow back. Massages improve your scalp and help improve hair growth. Remember the tight braids and tension is not suitable for the shaft of the hair because it only causes more shedding from the root and makes you more susceptible to alopecia.

NUBIA'S SIMPLE STEPS TO GROWTH:

1. Avoid the heat
   - Heat dries your hair out and can cause breakage.

2. Deep condition
   - This process should be done at least twice a month will help add more protein and moisture to your hair.
   (Be aware that too much protein for some may cause breakage).

3. Get a trim.
   - Some suggest every 6 weeks or a few times a year trimming your hair, but remember trimming does not cause your hair to grow faster.

4. Avoid harsh shampoos to cleanse your scalp.
   - Using a good chemical-free or organic cleanser helps keep your hair moisturized.
   - The ends of your hair doesn't require as much shampoo to cleanse.
   - It is recommended you shampoo every week, but some people wash every other day, which may impede your natural ability to produce oil.

5. Use liquid leave in conditioners.
   - They add vitamins especially vitamin B complex to help your hair grow.

6. Protect your ends.
   - Apply oils to the ends of the hair to help reduce splitting.

7. Drink plenty of water.

8. Reduce your stress
   - Try a new hobby.

9. Exercise
   - Yoga and inversion (positioning with feet up and head down) really helps improve the blood flow to your scalp.
   - Be careful; inversion is not good for everyone, especially for those who have medical problems.

10. Add Biotin to your vitamins regimen.
    - Biotin strengthens your hair and helps you retain your hair.
    - 1000 mg is recommended and can be purchased almost anywhere.

11. Be patient
    - Learn your hair care needs, relax, and watch it grow.

Health and medical conditions have an impact on hair growth. Your nutritional status, lack of hydration, and lack of iron in the blood affects hair. Anemia is one of the minor medical conditions that lead to weak, brittle, fragile hair . . . For healthy strong hair, you must have enough iron in your blood. Low iron is common in most African American women. Taking a prenatal vitamins regularly help with the iron deficiency. As you read the next section, I hope to give you a better understanding of why selecting vitamins to meet your needs is important for hair growth. Missing the most essential elements in your diet can affect not only hair growth but it can affect other medical conditions. In some cultures, hair growth is more prominent. I often find myself questioning what we eat that causes such hair growth.

We must explore iron levels in the blood stream because it is one of the most common deficits in African American women. After reviewing the facts about iron, you will understand why hair growth may be minimized. Fe or Iron is important in hair growth. African Americans' meal choices and consumption should have a daily nutritional balance that includes more protein, beans, and red meat. Iron is one of the few vitamins if taken alone that will not yield the full benefits of hair growth, because most people take it primarily to treat a medical condition. They fail to understand the nutritional requirements and the importance of keeping a healthy balance. Taking any single dose supplement like iron or Biotin is never the answer to hair growth, because single supplements alone does not absorb easily into the body. Iron-taking daily takes months before your body will build up enough iron hemoglobin for your red blood cells. I want you to look at each vitamin mentioned below so that you will understand why vitamins are necessary and important for your body. I recommend finding a good combination of vitamins in addition to a good diet. Take care of your body from the inside out, and you will find your natural journey an amazing transformation to a holistic way of living. Your blood requires enough oxygen, and good healthy cells develop and survive when enough oxygen is in our body. Focus on your health and your bodies requirements. Adding iron supplement will speed up the production of the Ferritin, which is a byproduct of the Iron. Iron is critical in cell growth and development as I mentioned before, you have to understand that iron produces so many other important factors in your body that are vital to growth and development of any cell. Anemia and thyroid conditions cause hair loss. There's many other medical condition that impacts your hair growth and loss so I suggest talking with your doctor. Make sure you are going for your yearly health screening and blood work.

Focus on good nutrition, drinking plenty of water, and maybe vitamins to help strengthen your hair. Growth is not determined by what you eat, but how your body responds to what you eat. Think of your hair strand as a living organism that maybe starving due to lack of the essential vitamins. Adding supplements are a great benefit if you are a vegetarian, on medications, pregnant, or have poor nutritional status. Spinach is an excellent source of iron, and it also has vitamin A and other great minerals the body needs for healing and repair.

Vitamin A is commonly found in your orange-colored fruits or vegetable like carrots, squash, sweet potato, apricots, and cantaloupe. Vitamin A is not just limited to the orange color, but liver, fish, and greens also provide a great source of Vitamin A. Most of us know Vit A is necessary for the retina, but it also plays a significant role in healthy hair and skin. There are other properties of the Vitamin A like the boosting effects on our immune function and rapid cell growth. Vitamin A alone is not a primary vitamin for hair growth, but its antioxidant properties aid in a healthy scalp and reduces thinning of the hair.[25]

Vitamin C acts as a hair growth booster and is found in oranges. Collagen is required to help build up elasticity to your hair. When combined with Vitamin C it helps with the absorption of the iron and enhances the synthesis of collagen. All fast growing cells and tissue repair require Vitamin C to speed up the process. Adding a little Vitamin C helps your body's immune response and is one of the keys to hair growth. Any deficiency in Vitamin C can result in hair loss and shedding. Vitamin C alone doesn't enhance hair growth, but in combination with other vitamins it will help increase your hair growth. Think healthy and be smart with all supplements.[1]

Vitamin D is crucial in the different phases of hair growth. The Anagen is the growing phase of our hair. Other phases of growth include the Catagen phase, which is the receding phase; and the Telogen or the resting phase of hair growth. Vitamin D is required to help our bodies go through this phases accurately. If we skip any phase of the hair growth cycle, it may cause poor development of our hair follicles and therefore yield in more shedding. Our bodies never get enough Vitamin D because we just don't get enough sunlight. Vitamin D is a precursor to all growth cycles, and the liver converts Vitamin D into Calcitrol. Our body needs Calcium and Calcitriol for the development of good strong, healthy hair. Vitamin D, Calcium, and Calcitriol controls and regulates the follicle to stimulate the cells. Without Vitamin D or any of the other essential elements the cells die and hair follicle dies. Try foods rich in Vitamin D include Salmon, eggs, tuna, mushrooms, milk, and other dairy products if you want to avoid taking an additional supplement. The vitamin D supplementation is extremely important if you suffer from chronic fatigue, weakness, and have aching muscles or if you suffer from chronic medical conditions that affect your bones, joints, or other autoimmune conditions.[8]

Vitamin B complex helps with our body's ability to deal with stress. B complex vitamins aid in hair growth. Remember, trauma and stress to your scalp need some Vitamin B to help it repair. Vitamin B12, Pantothenate, Vitamin B 5, and riboflavin, Vitamin B2 are produced from the B vitamin. Pantene is included in the hair care products and is found in Pantene. Panthenol is another type of Pantothenate, which is one of the B Vitamins. As you may know, the biotin is the best to help stimulate hair growth because it causes the follicle to be stronger, and it promotes cell growth. B complex includes B5, B7, B6, B12, B2 and they all aid in hair growth. You can take sublingual B supplements or try peanuts, watermelon, grapefruit, eggs, and more. Sublingual is simply any pill that goes under the tongue. Vitamin B is a critical supplement for anyone suffering from emotional integrity, and if you suffering from addictive behavior I strongly recommend B complex Vitamins. Alcoholics lack the B vitamins, and it is necessary to add the B vitamins including thiamine. Adding the Vitamin B supplements will slow down the shedding and help improve your emotional integrity.[9]

Protein or amino acid is a building block that helps with hormone regulations, blood cell growth, enzymes, antibodies, and new tissue. Protein replaces the old dead cells and produces new healthy cells. Eating meats and beans helps with protein imbalances.

Without protein, our hair will not grow. Your hair is protein, and there are multiple types of proteins. Lysine, Cystine, and Methionine are all-important factors to increasing protein for our hair to grow. Lysine helps our body transport the protein and other valuable chemicals to the hair follicle, which aid in the growth. Foods rich in Lysine are chicken, beef, and beans. All forms of Lysine like L-Cystine and L-Methionine contain Sulfur. Yes, chicken and beans are necessary for our hair. Sulfur is an antimicrobial agent that speeds tissue repair and helps our bodies make keratin. Keratin is simply the protein in our hair. Eating protein will help your hair recover and repair from any damage. Also try some beans and meats to help build up your protein. Our bodies require at least 70 grams of protein or more depending on your weight for cell growth. Check out your vitamin labels. Make sure you have enough protein to make your hair healthy and strong. Eating enough protein is always difficult, but adding a supplement may be necessary. There are other topical applications of protein like henna, keratin, and conditioners that can help you get some extra protein to build stronger hair. Be careful about adding too much protein to your hair, because it can increase shedding if you add too much protein. You can tell if you have added too much protein to your hair if you feel any hardening and dramatic texture changes in your hair.[15]

Vitamin K helps our body clot and also improves hair growth. Green leafy vegetables help with the clotting factors, and we must evaluate vitamins that contain Vitamin K and Vitamin A. Biotin, Vitamin D, and collagen together improve hair growth. Collagen is an amino acid or protein is required to build good healthy cells. Remember the goal is to have healthy hair. Other supplements and vitamins can help you with hair growth. Some people need to go to a dermatologist for more help because their medications, medical problems, and other issues cause them to lose their Hair. Sometimes to help with hair growth, Minovil may be necessary if all other methods fail. As a nurse, I find my stressful lifestyle impedes my hair growth. There just is no magical secret for hair growth when you are under so much stress. B vitamin supplements help, but you will need to reduce the stress and have a positive attitude. Finding a good hobby helps you deal with stress and also helps with hair growth, in addition to the use of some good supplements.

INVERSION

Inversion helps stimulate hair growth. Inversion methods are simple exercises or positioning when your head is positioned downward, position. This technique has been reported to increase growth to inches within seven days. Most people have never heard of the inversion method, although inversion techniques have been around for centuries. Through inversion blood flow is increased to the scalp, inversion improves hair growth; some people claim they noticed growth 1-4 inches within four months. Inversion is a yoga position when your feet are up in the air, and position the head downward. There are three different types of positions you can try one by placing the foot up against the with your head and neck will be flat on the ground, second position is when you are totally inverted upside down, and finally you can have your head downward like you are shampooing your hair in the sink. An inversion table can use be used also, but I strongly suggest talking with your doctor before trying any inversion exercises. Toxins released from the abdomen and blood flow affects your heart and other organs in your body. The third position is simply the position most people do when they wash their hair in the sink. Head down and feet remain on the ground. All methods of inversion should be avoided if you have serious conditions, any medical problems, are pregnant, or dizzy. Inversion also helps reduce the amount of gray hair. I strongly suggest you avoid inversion if you have any questionable concerns or medical condition.

MOISTURIZING SECRETS

Selecting the correct oil is imperative to hair growth. All oils are not created equally. Educate yourself on the different oils. Some oils are great for shine, some are better for growth, some oils help speed up the healing process, and some oils help improve the scalp. Try to avoid mixing too many oils together in the beginning of your journey to avoid potential risk that can occur to your hair and scalp. Always test your oil individually to avoid an allergic reaction or adverse effects.

Hair food is extremely important for hair, we must make sure to add a little to help reduce breakage. So many oils can be used to help the hair grow, and you have to find the perfect oil blend that works best for you, although I understand selecting to the best oil is complicated. Digestible oils work best for me, they are great for sleek and shine to my hair. Before investing in any oils, you must research the oils to make sure you find the best fit for your needs. Some oils are better for growth, itch relief, or some are great for fragrance, but not all oils are created equal. Organic oils really stimulates hair grow.

Rosemary oil is great for growth; it has other benefits for hair. It has a pleasant aroma and is known to delays the graying process of your hair. Rosemary leaves an invigorating feeling to the scalp with the tingling sensation. It stimulates the scalp and follicle which aides in growth and relieves itching.[27]

Peppermint oil adds great moisturizer that acts as an astringent that is commonly used to help the scalp by producing a tingling sensation. This oil may even help heal scalp problems like dandruff. Peppermint oil helps correct pH imbalances. Ph imbalances can cause a real problem with dryness.[5]

Jojoba oil is one of my favorite oils. Jojoba oil helps speeds up the healing process. This oil is very similar to the natural oil our scalp naturally produces. Jojoba does not spoil and mixes well to other oil combination. It is a great hydrator for the scalp. Jojoba oil adds elasticity, shine, and softens the hair. Jojoba oil seals, protects, and helps prevent further damage when heat is applied to the hair. Although jojoba oil is not cheap, a little bit can go a long way, and this oil is similar to your own natural oil. This oil is great for reducing frizz and unmanageable hair. Jojoba is a great hair growth stimulant. Try mixing it with avocado oil, coconut oil, and your favorite conditioner to do a deep conditioning treatment or pre-poo; and love the shine and softness of your hair. The use of this oil combination regularly for 6 months or greater you will notice a healthy head of hair.

Wheat germ oil is not commonly used oil for natural hair, but we must understand it has a great benefit for natural hair. Wheat germ is enriched with Vitamin E. It is a great in the prevention of cancer. I suppose you may be asking the question of why antioxidant or anti cancer causing properties in any hair care product is relevant. Hair, like the skin, is considered a living microorganism that grows rapidly. Any living cell growth is important; some cells are cancerous, and our body can develop tumors or cancer anywhere. The antioxidant properties in wheat germ are great to helps reduce the spread of unhealthy rapid growing cells to our head, brain, or scalp. Wheat germ also contains the Vitamin B, which is great for the stress response and also for poorly nourished cells that are rapidly growing in the scalp. Wheat germ helps with new cell development, and it helps promote rapid hair growth.[28]

Aloe Vera is an emergency 911 treatment. Aloe Vera is repairing oil. It is great for the repair of split ends. Apply oils to the end shaft and you will notice a big difference in growth and in the appearance of your ends. It can spoil, if discolorations are noticed. Purchase Aloe Vera in small amount for the best results. Aloe requires refrigeration. You can freeze it, but be cautioned that freezing the gel will change its gel form into a liquid, which may alter your styling aid. Aloe is great for repair of any damage, and helps reduce hair from falling out. It is a nice styling aide and makes the hair stiffen. For weather changes Aloe Vera will seal and protect the hair from winter damage. Aloe Vera has all kinds of vitamins and proteins that are great for growth. PH restoration from aloe will help you with growth and moisture. Aloe reduces scalp fungus and other potential pathogens from invading the scalp. Add a little aloe for your pre-poo, before shampooing and try adding wheat germ and coconut milk for a superb shine and seal.[6]

Kukui nut oil is oil similar to Noni. It is found in Hawaii. Kukui oil is rich in Omega 3 and is commonly mixed with Macadamia oil. It penetrates easily and it's soothing properties are normal utilized to help with sunburn, but it contains high levels of essential fatty acids like Linoleic and alpha. Linolenic oil absorbs easily into the skin and promotes tissue healing. Try this oil and you will notice significant changes in your skin and scalp if you suffer from any scalp disorder.[29]

Coconut oil is one of the most commonly used oils. It is readily available and inexpensive. Coconut oil is one of the few oils that changes its molecular structure and becomes a solid when cold. It adds more protection and seals your hair to prevent dryness during seasonal changes. Not only is it cheap, but also a little amount goes a long way. You don't have to worry about storage or spoiling as long as it is stored in a dark, cool, dry place. Thirsty, dull hair loves coconut oil because only a small amount is required for a brilliant shine. This oil may last for days. Most naturals refer to it as their hair care staple. Coconut oil works well for prepoo just a minimum amount or oil to the scalp and the ends of your hair before a shampooing. The preparation phase of washing your hair or pre-poo came from an ayurvedic secret of the

Indian culture. People of Indian use oils like coconut oil and Amla oil as a pre-poo. Amla is a bitter or sour fruit, which contains Vitamin C, which promotes the healing process. Ritualistic and cultural practices forbid any cutting of the hair. They are careful with their hair. Hot oil treatments enriched with coconut oil prevent moisturizing deficit. To prevent splitting and breakage try hot oil. African American women who wear their hair natural have adopted the idea to seal and protect the ends of the hair with the use of coconut oil to prevent breakage. It also reduces damage from the harmful process of shampooing. Coconut oil emulsifies for days. This oil is thick, and it stays on the hair shaft longer than any other oils because of it molecular structure. Coconut oil seals the cuticle to protect your hair during the hair washing. Split ends are common for everyone, and regularly clipping of the dead ends is necessary to keep the ends healthy and strong. Apply a small amount of coconut oil to the ends of your hair to prevent and reduce splitting.

Lavender oil is used for calming and relaxation traditionally. But lavender also nourishes the hair, adds a small amount of moisturizing to the scalp and strands, helps prevent shedding of the hair, improve the circulation, blood flow, and it also has antiseptic properties that reduce fungus, bacteria, microbes, dry scalp.[21]

Burdock root oil is great for scalp relief. Dandruff is a common problem, and the use of Burdock root improves the quality of the scalp. Burdock root helps with Vitamin A and fatty acids production. It is a like maple or molasses, and it is not recommended for people with allergies, diabetes, and if you are pregnant.[13]

Saw Palmetto—Through research for hair growth it has been determined that permanent hair loss is prevented by way of blocking certain hormone levels that trigger hair loss in the anagen stage. You can find this in the local Vitamin store or drug store. This plant is found commonly in California and the Atlantic coast. Saw Palmetto blocks the testosterone to DHT-dihydrotestosterone with cause's permanent alopecia. MSM is another supplement that helps improves hair growth by increasing the anagen phase of hair growth. So if you notice large areas where the hair is falling out, I recommend you talk with your doctor or pharmacist to see if there are any interactions prior to adding this supplement to help reduce the hair loss. Some people have noticed a significant difference in their hair loss after the use of Saw palmetto used topically. For oral use of the supplement, you will have to take Saw palmetto at least 2-3 months before you will notice a significant difference. And I will warn you that any vitamins supplement may potentially have effects on the liver, gallbladder, and the pancreas; so make sure you are communicating with your healthcare providers regularly.[14]

Stinging nettle has been around for centuries, and it works similar to the Saw Palmetto the hormone production of DHT. DHT blocks our follicles from absorbing protein which causes the hair to become frail and weak, causing and increase in shedding. Stinging nettle can be found in tea, vitamins supplement, or oil. Stinging nettle has been proven to reduce hair loss. Stinging nettle is also known as Utica Diocia. Try the Stinging nettle oil in your scalp at night and cover the head with a bonnet and cleanse the scalp in the morning. This is not one of the most pleasantly fragrant oil, I am not sure if you really want to go around smelling like this oil.[12]

Castor oil is my all time favorite oil because it adds humectants to the hair. People with low porous hair absorb moisture and shine to the hair nicely when castor oil is used. After applying castor oil, reapplication is not necessary for several days. Castor oil is rich in Omega 6, Vitamin E, essential amino acids. It really improves hair growth. Castor oil reduces common problems of the scalp like dandruff which is caused by fungus and bacteria. The hair will appear very shiny after the use of castor oil. Castor oil is very inexpensive, and it can be used indefinitely without any potential effects on your organ or health.[11]

I have done extensive research on flax seed oil and to tell you the truth I love the benefits of this oil. I make an oily butter-like gel out of the Flaxseed oil. Flaxseed is enriched in Omega 3, fatty acid alpha-linolenic acid. Flaxseed is not only beneficial for your hair, but it reduces cardiac disease, Diabetes, and lowering your cholesterol. Flax seed is well known for its antioxidant properties. These are one of the few oils that are a natural homeopathic. It has great benefits in the reduction in breast cancer and other cancers. Cancer growths are driven by the production of estrogen. Hormone levels off balanced caused so many health concerns from cancer, heart disease, stress, mental instability, and don't forget the aging process which creates a real concern for your hair also.

Flax seed oil. I absolutely love this oil because it is the oil that can be converted from seeds. Flax seed is rich in mega 3, Omega 6, ALA or alpha-linolenic acid which converts into the EPA – Eicosapentaenoic acid and DHA—Docosahexaenoix acid. Flax seed oil is as beneficial as fish oil. For hairstyling I love the gel that is formed out of the Flax seed. The gel formed by boiling hot water and strained the seeds into a clear gel with other oils like Aloe Vera and jojoba oil. Flax seed oil is great for shine and strengthens your hair.

Flax is not new to the industry; it has been around for centuries. Growth stimulation and healing properties to the inflamed scalp are great beneficial use of flax seed. Flaxseed is rich with B Vitamins, Magnesium, Potassium, Lection, Zinc, and Protein, Omega 3 and Omega 6, which shown great benefits in the treatment in ADHD and arthritis.

There are other benefits of flax seed. It helps lowers your blood sugar and has great benefits on your colon health. Try adding the seeds to your food, and you will notice a significant change in your bowel pattern. Flax seed lowers your risk of colon cancer.

Some companies are adding flax seed oil to their hair products for superior shine and growth to the hair. I make my own hair butter from the flax seed. I love the styling enhancements and the health benefits of the use of flax seed oil. Flax seed is very difficult to strain the seeds out of the mixture and produce the gel, but I have to say the rewards are so beneficial. I've noticed significant growth in my husband's thin areas of his head and my family has been using it for years. I, too, have a stress area in my hair, and I have noticed strengthening in the area. I also have a young girl I have been working with for about 6 months that had a lot of issues with dandruff and flaking. Her scalp has improved significantly. She was using Head and Shoulders and going to the dermatologist prior to coming to see me. To be honest, Head and Shoulders did not prevent her scalp problem. All the chemicals added to Head and Shoulder alters the benefits of the Zinc. I am not a doctor, but I am sharing my personal experiences and testimony with you.[16] Zinc is needed to heal your scalp.

Moroccan and Argan oil help reduce the frizz. Argan oil is found and produced through a very difficult process in Morocco. This oil is not produced in great volumes like other oils because of its limited tree sources. It adds great luster and shine to the hair and it is great for hair growth also. It has some antioxidant properties and also contains Vitamin E. It works a lot like the other oils in the prevention of scalp complication and dandruff. But both oils are very expensive and not produced in the United States. Be aware that most of these imported products contain preservatives. You will have and you will have to pay a larger price to purchase 100% authentic Moroccan oil or Argan oil which may or may not be as potent by the time it reaches you in the United States. It has been said that anyone with 3c hair type (which is loose, softly coil hair) up to 4 hair type, (which is hard and has a tight coil to a coarse) may not get the full benefits from the use of either oils because the oil doesn't not always works for all hair types. True Argan oil has little to no scent and has to be stored in a cool dark place. I venture to say that by the time its gets to the US or your house it may not be as beneficial as you think.[10]

Olive oil is an easy, readily available, and can be found almost anywhere. Olive oil works well for some people, but it is not growth-guaranteed oil. Although olive oil is available everywhere, it is Mediterranean oil, and it has been used for centuries. This oil is high in fats. Olive oil repairs and invigorates the scalp by keeping it moisture. It works well in the prevention of split ends, and it is relatively inexpensive. Olive oil has antioxidant properties, and it is commonly used for sensitive hair. This oil is great for hair in so many ways because it is lightweight, and this emollient contains Vitamin E.[3]

Grapeseed oil contains Linoleic, Oleic, and Stearic, Palmitic, Myristic, and Lauric. Myristic is a crystalline fatty acid, it is digestible and non-toxic. Oleic is common found in Emu oil it is a monounsaturated Omega-9 fatty acid, it can be found in animals and plants also. Linoleic is an Omega 6, and it is also known as the carboxylic acid, it is an essential fat. Palmitic is a fatty acid found from animals and some plants. Lauric acid is known to kill bacteria, virus, and fungus and it may be found in other oils like coconut oil. It is an essential fatty acid that is light, odorless, and can be used as a mild astringent.

Amla oil is commonly used in Indian hair. This oil strengthens the hair from the inside to the outer core of the hair. Normally women prepare or pre-poo the hair the night before by applying the Amla oil to the entire head. This oil is not a pleasant in fragrance, but it adds great protein and moisture balance to the hair. Upon awakening in the morning, you will have to shampoo the hair. Some African women have noticed no benefit to this treatment and some have report the combination of the Amla oil and their conditioner to cause more shedding, so I would have to say you must be aware of combinations of different oils and protein may alter the effect of what you are hoping to accomplish with the Amla oil.

Avocado oil is great oil for hair growth, it adds nutrients, and vitamins to help you obtain a healthy scalp. I have a home hair care regimen I use to help me get the best benefit out of avocado oil. Try the avocado mask to help improve your hair growth today.

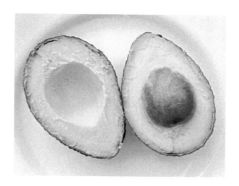

Avocado Hair Mask

1 small avocado mashed

1 spoon plain Greek yogurt

½ spoon of honey

Add oil of your choice

Mix all the ingredients to a creamy paste. Section off your hair and apply evenly. Make sure to massage your scalp to penetrate the mask for at least 10 minutes. Cover with your plastic cap. Let the mask sit for 30 minutes to 1 hour. Sit under the dryer or allow your natural body heat to allow your scalp to absorb the oil from the mask. Rinse in the shower, dry, and style as normal. Your hair will feel soft, shiny, and moisturized.

This mask is great for protein restoration. It contains over 20 vitamins and minerals to your scalp or skin. This Mexican fruit is fortified with Lutein, which is great for the eyes, antioxidants, Alpha carotene, Beta-carotene, and Zeaxantin. The benefits of the oils produce from the avocado are richer than our traditional almond, olive, and safflower oil.

Shea butter adds shine and healing properties to both your hair and skin. It can be purchased in bulk at a low price. The Shea nut is found in Africa and it is great for soothing the scalp, sealing moisture to the scalp, and protection from the UV rays. It softens the hair and helps reduce fragile and brittle hair from breaking. It also has some great effects on the aging process because of its dermatological repairing effects. Try a nice compressed refined Shea butter and Coconut oil. It is definitely one of the most popular and inexpensive oils on the market. This oil is considered to be hydrophobic. Hydrophobic is defined as the separation of oil and water into two components; the coconut oil repels the water and prevents the hair from drying. Coconut oil is the most commonly used component or ingredient when doing a pre poo. Pre Poo is simply a preparation phase before shampooing the hair. To prepare for the cleaning you will saturate the end of the hair with oil prior to shampooing. Coconut repels water, which makes it hydrophobic oil. I love it because of its benefits to low porous hair and the humectants effects. Coconut oil before shampooing actually helps the hair follicle swell and absorb more protein, water molecules, and moisture, which help in reducing splitting and breakage. A little coconut oil goes a long way, and I encourage you to try coconut oil to improve the moisture and hydration balance of your hair. Avocado oil helps with growth, shine, and reduces lice, fungus, and other bacteria caused by poor hygiene.

Neem oil is another Indian oil that is used as a pesticide. It is widely found in Asia, and it is bitter and used as an astringent to promote healing, it purifies the blood by detoxification the liver. This oil also has great benefits in hair use in that it grows the hair and has great healing properties for the scalp. It aids a great shine, and it is good for the treatment of lice, fungus, bacteria, and other germs that invade the scalp. The smell is very pungent, and most people that use the oil use it at night and wash it out in the morning. This oil's stench is compared to burnt peanut butter and much worse than Sulfur. Try this oil if you have experienced scalp irritations and if your hair growth has been impeded by scalp problems.

Vitamin E oil is healing oil, and it is used for dermatological problems. Vitamin E oil is essential for repair, and it aids in growth by way of the skin or scalp repair. Vitamin E can be found in several of the oils mentioned above, and I would recommend adding this oil to your hair care regimen if you have had any scarring or surgical repair of the head.

There are many more oils like Rosemary, Peppermint, Tea Tree, Geranium, Marjoram, Cedarwood, Lavender, and more. You must find the best oil that works for your hair and finding the right combination will help promote your hair growth. I have my favorite blends, and I hope that my recipes and combinations will be a great guide for you. I will have to say starting off with a little coconut oil is a great option. I started my journey with 100 % pure unrefined Shea butter and found that most of the product combinations mixed with Shea butter produces lots of builds up, white flakes, and just did not mix well with all oils. Explore and try different oils to determine the staple that works best for you. Continue to read and you will find additional growth aids that will help improve your hair strength and enhance your hair growth.

Drinking plenty of water is very critical in hair growth. We exposure our body and hair to harmful chemicals, medication, and environmental factors: that is why it is critical for us to flush our bodies of the toxin, by drinking plenty of water. Vitamins that include biotin, Vitamin C, Vitamin D, Vitamin E silicone, collagen, Zinc, are helpful to the growth of your hair. I recently started drinking Jell-O to help with the elasticity of my hair. Protein is essential for growth also, so eat a nice balance meal include your meat or your eggs. Supplements may also be required to help you with your nutritional deficits that may cause stunted hair growth.
Other alternative hair growth secrets that have been used for centuries can be found in your own garden or kitchen.

TOP INGREDIENTS FROM YOUR HOME OR GARDEN

Aloe Vera juice or gel—is an emollient and is perfect for sealing the moisture in your hair.

Avocado or banana mask—repairs damage hair and leaves your hair silky and super moist—contains complex Vitamin A, B, C, E, K.

Eggs—protein for healing also contains B12 and Sulfur.

Vegetable glycerin—acts as strong humectants (binds to water molecules).

Coffee or black tea rinse—caffeine acts as a stimulant to bind with the conditioner.

Green tea-also stimulates the follicles and reduces hair loss and contains Vitamin C, D, E and Pantheon or B5.

Coconut oil—seals moisture in your hair.

Olive oil—full of antioxidants that repairs and nourish dry damage hair.

Flax seed—moisturizes and is perfect for styling without damaging your hair, also enriched with Omega 3 and Linseed.

Vinegar—improves your ph balance (2.8—3.0) also acts as a natural antibiotic.

HEALTH BENEFITS

There are a multitude of reasons for going natural. A great percentage of women transition to natural because they want to improve the quality of their hair, but there are health benefits for letting go of the man made process chemicals. Some health reasons women go natural are they have no other option such as when they are undergoing cancer treatment. The cancer treatment causes hair loss and not the disease itself. Chemotherapy and radiation attacks rapidly new growth of the cell. Hair cells grow rapidly. After chemo treatments the hair will grow back, so do not fear the hair will come back. According to chemotherapy.com the hair loss begins within 2-3 weeks of treatment and is restored within 2-3 months after chemotherapy. Shave your legs; within 2 days you will notice a great amount of hair growth, so don't be afraid if you are going through chemotherapy, just understand your hair will grow back.

Stress also plays an important role on hair growth and hair loss. Hair loss is really determined by so many different factors like a healthy mind and body. Hair loss can be totally devastating to women. You must know that hair lost that turns to baldness is known as alopecia. Alopecia is a complete loss of hair and this may be temporary or permanent. Alopecia is commonly caused by genetic factor that cannot be changed, try a better diet and exercise may enhance your hair growth. Remember just because momma was a diabetic and had hypertension it does not mean you have to have the same medical condition. I like to focus on primary and secondary prevention because a healthy lifestyle can change the makeup for predisposition and alter your outcome. There are some diseases that cause hair loss like Diabetes, thyroid, anemia, Asthma, autoimmune diseases, and Alzheimer's disease.

I know science and medical research will say I have taken it to the extreme to say Asthma can cause hair loss. Well let me break it down for you. Asthma is a condition where people are deprived oxygen; if you have been left without oxygen for long time healthy cells die. Medical science has proven that the use of medications like steroids definitely cause lots of hair loss, but lack of oxygen causes the slowing down of good healthy cell growth. So I say if you have any medical condition in which you are under close guidance of a doctor and you are taking medications as prescribed, be aware of the effects on your hair and know that supplements may help reduce some of the hair loss.

Thyroid creates hormones that have a direct correlation to the antigen stage of your hair growth. Thyroid conditions cause shedding and hair loss. You must seek a medical profession for any questions about hair loss. Shedding is normal at times but if the shedding created areas of baldness you need to get blood work to determine what deficiencies you may be having.

Diabetes affects hair growth because of the medications, large amount of sugar, and stress. Any stress to the body will cause the hair to fall out. Think about the Fight or Flight Syndrome our bodies; when the body is under stress the hair sticks up to attention, and if your parasympathetic and sympathetic nervous system is at alert for too long your body will react and hormones will be released, this causes death to your hair and cause great amounts of hair loss. Good nutrition and avoidance of too much sugar and carbohydrates is necessary for growth or hair retention. Too many carbohydrates can affect your hair growth and some people have gluten allergies and the gluten allergy will cause the hair to shed and even cause baldness. If you notice scalp irritations, sores, and baldness please don't avoid it get it checked out and also think about possible allergies triggers irritations.

Some chemicals you use to chemically straighten the hair can cause fibroid tumors or cancer. There are other illnesses that cause alopecia. Examples are HTN, DM, thyroid condition, Alzheimer's, and other medical problems. People have to take extra precautions to protect their hair loss and alopecia. But I want you to understand that it is not just the medical problems and the medication that can cause the hair loss; it may be just the darn chemicals you apply to your scalp.

Relaxers cause uterine fibroids, brain tumors, and cancer. It is not uncommon for black women to have hysterectomy by the ages of 45 because of the uterine fibroids. Fibroids grow early as women begin their cycle when we expose our young daughters to chemical containing lye. Alteration begins from the scalp from the chemical attacks the brain and the hormones.

The pain begins and you are fooled by that old saying, 'no pain, no gain'. Was it worth it to straighten your daughter's hair, and now she is complaining every month about the horrendous cramping and pain? No one ever told you the perm was the big contributor to her sharp pain. After years go by the damage is done there is nothing you can do to change, not even stop chemically relaxing your hair. Perms can affect your fertility and sex drive. I always thought it was taboo that you should not perm when pregnant; it was true! I can only assume the chemicals may be passed on to the unborn child, so really it was not even necessary for your child to even have a perm to inherit those dreadful fibroids. Chemicals are Chemicals people! We need to wise up about what we subject our temple to. A little research will prove this theory; among women that do not perm the hair during childbirth, some females are less susceptible to fibroids and uterine cancer. The fibroids are precancerous and grow like a large tumor in your body, and the chemicals we expose ourselves to are just not worth the silky-straight hair. Perms do affect our hormone levels. I am a testimony to this fact. I had my second child and my hair was long and straight. I had one of the celebrity stylists in Atlanta (who did the hair of the singing group TLC) doing my hair. Well right after I had the baby my hair started shedding in a vast amount and I was super concerned. I went back to her weeks after the birth of my son for some kind of emergency deep conditioning treatment, and she told me there was nothing she could do: the hormones and the chemicals in my hair just did not agree. I was mad as a wet hen! We use the term "over processing" so much we think it was the stylist's fault. Well guess what baby; it was that darn perm that caused my hair to shed in patches. God never meant for you to alter the ph of your hair. Hair ph is normally low and acidic, but man got wise and changed the ph to an alkaline state. Alkaline state requires a ph balancing and correction. Remember when your grandmother would tell you to get the vinegar to correct or reverse the problem? Well, I think granny was definitely right. Vinegar is acidic and reduces the effects of over process hair. Transform your naps or kinks to a healthy head of hair. Honestly once your hair damage is done; the use of acid or vinegar just will not fix the damage.

Did you know there are benefits to that caustic chemical? Yes, when caustic chemicals burn, we generally think of acids, but bases can burn also. Perms are caustic and they alter the effect of the hydrogen and the ph and it may have some benefits. People use the perm to burn out and dry the head sores, but the scalp damage and growth problems will occur after the application of that perm. I guess after you have already lost hair and the unsightly bald patch is there you might consider anything to get that hair back and to kill the invasion or sore to the scalp.

Because I am a medical professional, it is my duty to educate you about the facts of the chemicals. Now people have this unconcealed notion that the other straighteners are good. Keratin treatments contain formaldehyde, and you need to wise up about putting everything on your hair. Let me explain it simply; once any chemical is applied it is attached to your hair until it is cut out. People go 6-9 months without chemicals and assume the chemical is out, but they are wrong; the chemicals stay in your hair until it grows out completely or it all falls out. If you don't believe me, then I advise you to feel the ends of your hair. If the ends are not curly or feel different from the hair closest to your scalp, then you definitely still have relaxed ends. You don't get rid of those harmful chemicals once it is there; you have to live with it until it is cut off, or until you lose all of your hair.

There are so many chemicals that cause medical problems that you just have not been told about, and I want to make sure you are aware that the junk you use is going to harm you in some way. Even our men have major medical problems later in life; scientific research needs to explore the link between Afro-American men and the prostate cancer. Texturizers potentiate African American prostate cancer in men. Men should try to avoid any hair care product that mimic the estrogen like Bisphenol. Any products that contact the phthalates can alter the sperm and the reproductive system. This is only my theory and I hope people understand that chemicals can cost us our life. The risk of beauty should never cost you your life. Let go of the cancerous chemicals, embrace the gray, and embellish your imperfections.

My company's logo is "Transform your Nappy to Happy". Nappy is good and not our traditional thinking of course, kinky and "bad hair". There is no such thing as bad hair, as Chris Rock said himself. According to the Webster dictionary, nappy is kinky. The urban dictionary defines nappy as a state of coiling, unprocessed hair. Transform yourself from nappy to happy because God never intended any offense in you creating your nap.

TO SHAMPOO OR NOT

Black women traditionally never thought they could wash in go. Now naturals all over have discovered the secrets of wash and go. I am embarrassed because my mother never taught me how to wash my hair. At the age of 12, my mother told me I was on my own and it was time for me to wash my thick mane. I washed my hair in a circular motion, as though I was in the Herbal Essence commercials back in the 70-80's, and caused my hair to kink, snap, and pop. I had to define my shampooing technique without causing more breakage and damage. People seem to believe the care of thick hair requires too much time, and feel it is difficult to wash, detangle, and go. Today women wearing their hair natural wash it, and in minutes they are ready to go. Fresh, clean smelling hair only requires the right shampoo and oil balance. You should never just wash your hair in a circular motion, which creates kinks and matting of the hair. There are several great washing techniques for coarse thick hair, by simply creating your hands spread out and pulling the fingers close together, by grabbing the scalp inward toward your fingers. Gentle massage to the scalp doesn't have to cause the ends to get matted and tangled. Wash from the scalp to the ends and keep it simple just focus on the scalp then rinse thoroughly. If your hair is unmanageable, high porous hair, unable to get to the scalp because your hair is too thick, try braiding the hair into 4 sections prior to washing so that you can focus on the scalp and have less tangling of the ends of your hair. Just braid your hair in 4 sections, focus primarily on the scalp and cleanse very carefully. Handle your hair with care, and you can avoid the hair trauma created by shampooing of your hair.

The most common question naturals face today is, "What cleansers do you use?" All shampoos purchased out of the store contain some type of preservative. Preservatives are not great for our hair. Try to avoid shampoos containing Sulfate, Laureth Sulfate, and Cocamide: they are the foaming agent in the shampoos, which causes cancer. They are great for super lather and suds, but not great for your hair. Substitute your shampoos for African black soap.

Cocamide DEA has been proven to cause Cancer. Cocamide is a derivative of coconut which makes foam and for shampoos and body wash. The FDA has just produced a list of the effects of the shampoos containing cocamide, and you must learn to read the labels before attempting to use these products. Shampoos that contain more cocamide are: Paul Mitchell, Palmolive, Soft n Pretty, Crème of Nature, Doo Gro, Design Essentials, American Crew . . . For more information please go to the Center for Environmental Health or ceh.org.

Other product stabilizers and form boosters to be aware of that cause cancer are Cocamide, MEA, and DEA—Cetyl Phosphate, DEA oleth-3 Phosphate, Lauramide DEA, Linoleamide

MEA, Myristamide DEA, Oleamide DEA, Stearamide MEA, TEA—Lauryl Sulfate, and Triethanolamine. FDA has recently posted this information, and you need to be aware of cancer causing agents. Again a natural way of life includes avoidance of preservatives and other unavoidable hazardous factory made and produces chemicals. Read your labels or try mixing your own products.

Sodium Laurent Sulfate—This chemical is known to be cancer causing or carcinogenic, and you will find this is in a variety of shampoos. The FDA has recently posted multiple warnings about this foam-aiding chemical in the shampoos because of its great risk and potential problems for your skin and eyes.

Methylchloroisothiazolinone is one of the worst kinds of preservatives. This additive makes the products last longer on the shelf and reverses the good effects of the products. You will not only find it in your hair care products, but you may find it in your cosmetics also. It has been banned and restricted in some areas across the United States.

Ammonium Chloride is not digestible and may cause eye irritations. It may cause serious damage to your respiratory tract if inhaled.

Propylene Glycol is a great moisturizer and used for your GI tract, but it is harmful to your respiratory system and has been linked to disorders and autoimmune problems in children.

Strong Fragrance or Perfumes—are really not good in any way. They do cause serious allergic reaction and add no benefits to your hair.

Recently, Jacelyn Baer (a white lady) admitted to the world that she stopped washing her hair in the traditional way with shampoos over 5 years ago. Her hair looks healthy and strong. I bet she feels better than she has ever felt before since she gave up the unhealthy chemicals. Taking the organic approach to hair care yields to a healthier balance in your home and lifestyle. I wonder her reason for avoiding the shampoos. A lot of naturals go natural for health and for problems with low porosity; which leads to drying, lack of elasticity, and lots of shedding. Shedding becomes a greater problem for women who have low porous hair. Looking at the results of Jacelyn avoiding the harmful shampoos, her hair is stronger and appears healthier. Jacelyn claims she does wash her, not traditionally with the use of shampoo, she said her hair care regimen consist of the use of baking soda and vinegar. These two cleansing aides are both natural and they also don't destroy your hair, if balanced properly. I have to commend Jacquelyn for sharing that she has gone shampoo free. She expressed concern, "for paraben, phthalates, petroleum, byproducts, and other dangerous chemicals are not good for your hair."

African Americans are not the only ones who benefit from an organic approach hair care. I hope Jacelyn's shared story improves your reviews about your hair care universally.

The use of oils regularly helps cleanse the hair because oil exfoliates and also removes dead layers to help improve the scalp. I challenge you to wash your body regularly with baby oil; watch layers of skin, and dirt fall off. Take the oil challenge and see if the results increase the skin elasticity, and improve the texture of your hair. Oil improves all aspect of our beauty, appearance, and it is naturally produced in our bodies. Serum is the natural oil in our body. So never be afraid to cleanse your hair with oil or try a pre-poo method before cleansing your hair. The greatest benefit of going natural is clean and fresh. Some people wear braids for 4 weeks or longer without cleaning their scalp; this is not a good hygienic practice. Clean hair is critical. Think about your intimate pleasure when a man kisses, caresses your neck, and smells the sweet smell of your clean fresh hair. The pleasure increases from the scent of the women holistically and it is nice for him to run his hands through fresh smelling hair! Keep your hair clean, and avoid the flakes. Make your hair a delightful part of your body! Use fragrances and other natural oils to give your hair some better balance. Big hair is sexy, and clean hair is even more appealing.

Like a virgin is untouched or not easily stimulated by anything and anyone, virgin hair is hair in its unaltered or original state. Your hair doesn't like all kind of products! Some hair is resistant to the penetration of chemicals. Keep hair care simple! If you are new to the transitioning and you really are confused about the how to maintain the virgin hair you must study and do your research. I love the YouTube videos because they offer great guidance for styling, product reviews, and growth tips. Try avoiding the unrealistic conception that your results will be exactly the same as someone. Love to embrace your hair. We all are created equal but unique. Some Mediterraneans grow their hair at a more rapid rate, have stronger follicles, and due to genes they retain their hair length. I thought if I could just eat what they eat and care for my hair the way they do I would be able to get the same hair length. Well that only sets us up for hair care failure. We are always looking for that magic potion to get the maximum growth. I remember shampooing my knots and trying to detangle a real mess. I thought the use of olive oils was the key to growth and shine, but for some olive oil may be the answer for their hair. But for me olive oil was not the definitive answer for my hair. I just did not know what to do with my hair in its natural state. I needed a solution to my virgin hair and just did not know what to do with it. Virgin hair requires very basic instructions. Like a baby that has just been born, it needs tender loving care. Start off with a simple regimen for about 4-6 weeks, and try not to mix any chemicals or go from product to product, because you will never ever get the full benefits until you understand how different products works. I love coconut oil and it is one of the best moisturizer and humectants. Although I love it I have had a mild reaction when eating too much raw coconuts with skin bumps. I continue to use it because it works so well. I don't have hair down my back, I get more shedding than most, and also noticed coconut oil does not mix well with other styling products I use. I don't get the flakes in the scalp, but I get product build up in the hair when I use styling products. My daughter says "Yuk! You need to wash those nasty white balls out of your hair!" I'm learning that too much product weighs the hair down, and causes more breakage for those people that have low porosity hair or lack of elasticity (ability to stretch). I generally use heavy products for styling only rarely, but I avoid wearing the heavy products for no more than 3 days because it has to be washed out. My hair does not absorb much oil or water, so I have to wash it out due to the product build up. Virgin hair care is simple and not that complicated. A weekly washing, little oil, detangle nightly braids, a satin scarf, wake up in the morning rub a little oil take the braids out, use a rat tale pick to lift the roots up, then leave your hair allow for the rest of the day and repeat nightly. You need an extra pomade barrier or something to give you a glossy or shiny look, before applying your favorite styling product. Keep in mind, products may cause build up or cake up and require more frequent cleaning. Just try to avoid the use of too many products in the beginning of your journey, until you have discovered your hair care staple. Your staple is what we refer to as your must-have products. Remember to read all labels and be aware that some of the chemicals can harm your hair, and remember to set realistic about your hair goals for your hair. The more you apply tension by the tight styles, the more breakage you may notice.

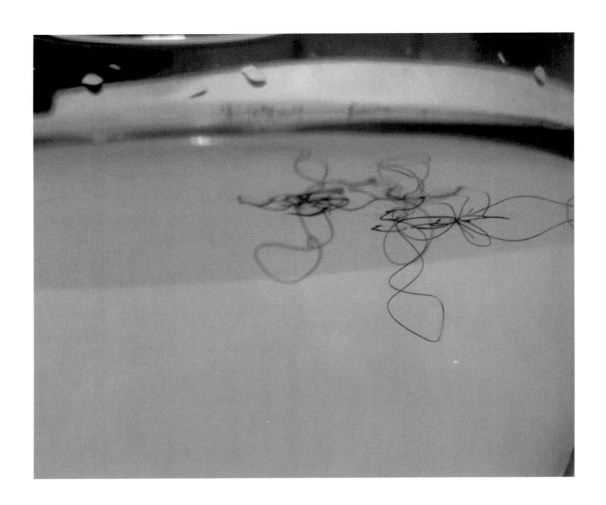

POROUS TESTING

To determine if you have high porous versus low porous hair, I recommend you get a clear glass of water, and put some of your clean hair that sheds into a glass of water. If there is any product on the hair this simple test will not be accurate, so make sure the hair is clean and free of any product. Allow the hair to set into the water for at least 40-60 sec, and if the hair goes to bottom of the water that means your hair is high porous. The hair that floats is low porous hair which means the hair may appear shiny and healthy, but product and water doesn't penetrate very easily. This hair really is more susceptible to breakage and destruction.

Low porous hair is simply a problem with hydration and moisture balance. This hair lacks elasticity and is easy to break. I avoided deep conditioners and protein because I never notice a difference in my hair. Low porous hair simply does not require the protein because it is full of protein. The cuticles are tightly compressed together and resist any water or oil from going into the cuticle. The best solution for low porous hair is to spray with water and then oil it. Daily spray of water will help reduce the tension to the hair and improve your ability to make other moisturizing products to seal the cuticles. Think about oil in water. If water is present, the oil is more prominent and it seals the hair shaft. Coconut, glycerin, Aloe Vera, and steam conditioning are really helpful. Find other humectants products that will help your hair maintain both the moisture and hydration. The key idea about your porosity is to balance hair care needs (medium not too high or low porous hair). Your hair will feel soft, and you will notice less breakage when you apply your favorite hair care product and oils. Your hair will not be dry and will absorb the products. High or low porous hair can be altered into medium porous hair, which is the goal.

I've noticed in the past that some people chemically process or dye their hair to open the cuticles enough to allow the moisture and protein to adhere to the hair for easier styling. Really finding a more organic solution to porosity problems is a better option. Dyeing and applying a chemical can cause permanent imbalances to the hair follicle and therefore yield more hair loss. The best solution again is trying water and then oil if your hair is not high porous. If the hair is high porous the hydration and moisture is not a real problem.

High porous hair on the contrast has the cuticles more open. This hair is dull looking and needs more oil and protein to keep the cuticles from falling out. Styling is less complicated and the hair is more flexible. Moisturizing shampoo, aloe Vera mixtures, and hydrolyzed protein is the best solution for this type hair. Again protein, conditioners are the best solution for the high porous hair.

Dandruff is a real problem that people have, and as a natural it may worsen especially if you are not properly caring for your scalp. Dandruff is those god-forsaken flakes that make your scalp itch. Dandruff is like a bug, a pest that gets out of control. Some people confuse product build—up with the dandruff flakes of the scalp. Product build-up is generally on the hair not in the scalp, but settles on the hair shaft and they are very sticky.

Some dandruff is a result of inflammatory response, and some dandruff is not caused by any inflammatory reaction. Growing dandruff is mild and easy to eliminate by good scalp washing and massage. Blocked oil glands can also cause dandruff, and exfoliation is necessary to help unclog the scalp. *Head and Shoulders* is and has been the most common treatment for dandruff, but so many people tell me it just does not work. People have tried yogurt, vinegar, coffee, tea tree, Listerine, and other non-traditional treatments to eliminate the nasty appearance and itch of the scalp from dandruff. These nontraditional therapies really work well, and you must understand that the root cause of any dandruff is simple; it may be an inflammation, infection, or fungus. Sounds disgusting, but fungus invades our bodies from the head to the inside of the mouth and stomach, and our feet.

Fungus is a problem cause from many sources. Our diet has a major role in fungal growth. Eating too much sugar or carbohydrates will increase the risk for fungus. Poor hygiene is another issue but not really a common cause of fungal scalp. Some people whose hair holds on the water into the scalp trigger fungus. Shampooing weekly and the use of oil will help heal your scalps appearance. This is common for hair that is slow drying and very thick. Water is trapped and it sits on the scalp. Head fungus is avoidable by just simply drying the scalp and allowing air to get to the scalp. Now remember, if you scratch all the time you open up small lesions and skin irritations, so no matter what you do the scalp will become irritated and not heal. Commercial products and shampoos really don't help with dandruff. You may want to go to a dermatologist to get more help with treating scalp problems and dandruff. One nontraditional treatment is to dilute Listerine with water and spray to your scalp. Leave this treatment on for 10 minutes then wash it out. Listerine is a very powerful antiseptic because it kills germs. Studies have shown that over 76 % of the people that used the Listerine treatment to kill the dandruff or Bottle Bacillus had great success at correcting the problem.

Tea tree oil is great for the treatment of scalp problems. Tea tree has antimicrobial properties that have been linked to reducing and killing all types of infections especially fungus. It may burn and sting a little when you apply it so I highly suggest you avoid this if you have openings wounds in your scalp. The smell is a little pungent. The smell can be corrected by adding the tea tree oil to your favorite shampoo. Tea tree is not limited to the outside of your body it can also be used in your mouth, it is relatively safe.

Monistat to the scalp is also a treatment women have resorted to for treatment of scalp problems and itch. Monistat kills the yeast in the private are also works great for other areas have been attacked by fungus. Fungus really is not easy to correct, it takes time and patience to correct. Stick with the treatment plan to correct it and I believe it will take over one month to know if the therapy is going to work for you.

Ph restorative treatment is also another way to help correct growth, dandruff, and irritations of the scalp I recommend using a ph balanced shampoo to help correct scalp problems and restore the hair to improve growth and reduces shedding.

Exploring different shampooing techniques will help you determine the best option for cleaning your hair. I find that sectioning off the hair in 4 works great for the reduction of tangles and it also allows me to really focus on the scalp for the best cleaning. Pre-poo is a great cleansing tech. Pre-poo is preparing your hair for the shampooing, by the use of oils saturation to the ends of the hair prior to a washing to keep the cuticles sealed during the shampooing. This method is great for sealing the bonds of the hair to prevent breakage and splitting of the ends during the shampooing. The friction from the shampooing can cause more damage than careful combing and detangling. The best pre-poo sealers are the olive oil or the coconut oil because they repel water molecules and protect and seal the hair.

Co-wash is simply using conditioner to wash the hair. Both techniques are equally important to maintaining strong hair and protecting your hair from breakage. Co-washing is a simply way to avoid the tangles and help replenish the ends of your hair with oil and moisture. After a co wash your hair should look and feel fabulous.

I hope you understand the importance of products you select to pamper your mane. I have already forewarned you of the importance of avoiding certain shampoos. Because of the health effects they produce. But I want you to know that you there are healthier options for cleaning your hair, and you have to read the labels before applying any man-made factory produces to your hair. All products sold on the self have to have some kind of preservative to keep it on the shelf and to keep it from spoiling. Spoilage is very common in products with aloe vera, and you have to be careful because it may lose it potency if it is past the expiration date. I do not recommend you get any shampoo in bulk; the smaller quantities really are best for you. Pure African black soap last a long time, but when you start mixing it with other products and water you will notice mold or fungus growth if you do not use it in a timely manner. Keep all hair products in a cool dry place and try not to mix large amounts; only use what you need for each cleaning, and you will find that your hair and scalp will look much healthier. Here is the list of products on the FBA warning list:

UPDATE: Companies with products shown in green have already committed to CEH in writing that they will reformulate their products, without cocamide DEA.

PRODUCT	BRAND NAME	COMPANY	RETAILER
Classic clean shampoo (for all hair types)	Prell	Ultimark Products	Walgreens
Medicated Conditioning Shampoo	MG217	Lake Consumer Products	Rite Aid
Daily Shampoo	American Crew Classic	American Crew	CVS
Olive Oil Shampoo	Organics by Africa's Best	House of Cheatham	CVS
Caprice (Acti-Ceramidas Shampoo)	Palmolive	Colgate-Palmolive Co.	FoodMaxx
Mane 'n Tail Shampoo	Straight Arrow	Straight Arrow Products	FoodMaxx
Climate Control Defrizzing Shampoo	Ouidad	Ouidad Products	Sephora
TUI (moisturizing sulfate-free shampoo)	Carols Daughter	Carols Daughter Products	Sephora
Brilliance Shampoo	Rusk	Rusk	CVS

Kid's Bubble Bath (Bubble Gum Scent)	Little Ones/Kmart	Kmart	Kmart
Classic Herbal Essence Shampoo (all hair types)	Vanart	Made by Estilo Y Vanidad, Distributed by Midway Importing	Kmart
Therapeutic Anti-Dandruff Shampoo	TopCare	Neutrogena Corporation	Lucky
Cleanse Hydrating Shampoo	BIOSILK	Farouk Systems	Lucky
Maximum Strength Medicated Dandruff Shampoo	Equate	Wal-Mart	Wal-Mart
Awapuhi Ginger Shampoo	Organix	Vogue International	CVS
"Ricitos de Oro" Chamomile Baby Shampoo	Grisi	Unknown	Walgreens
Cabellino Shampoo Chile Con Romero	Grandall	Grandall Dist. Co	Kmart
Dandruff Shampoo Selenium Sulfide	Image Essentials	Kmart	Kmart
Nutress Hair Protein Pack Treatment Shampoo	Nutress Hair	Nutress Hair	Glamour Beauty Supply
Treatment Curly Hair Moisturizing Shampoo Keratin and Cupuacu Butter	nuNAAT	nuNAAT	Glamour Beauty Supply
Luxury Care 3 Plus Frizz Control Shampoo	Luxury Care	Lustrasilk	Glamour Beauty Supply
Anti Breakage Neutralizing Shampoo Gel	Mega Growth	Strength Of Nature	Glamour Beauty Supply
Tea Tree Special Shampoo	Paul Mitchell	John Paul Mitchell Systems	Glamour Beauty Supply
Plant Extracts & Moroccan Argan oil Dry, Itchy Scalp Shampoo Controls Dandruff	At One With Nature	BioCare Lab	Glamour Beauty Supply
Gentle Cleansing & Conditioning Shampoo Aromatic Natural Essences pH balanced	Calm Cleanse	Johnson Products Co.	Glamour Beauty Supply
Hair Polisher Shampoo with "Sparkle Lites"	Fantasia	Fantasia Industries	Glamour Beauty Supply
African Essence Neutralizing Shampoo Plus Proteins and Conditioners	African Essence	Universal Beauty Products	Glamour Beauty Supply
VIA Natural Style Moisturizing Shampoo	VIA	Universal Beauty Products	Glamour Beauty Supply
Fair Trade Honey Shampoo	Lush	Lush	Lush
Sunflower & Coconut Detangling Conditioning Shampoo	Crème Of Nature	Colomer USA	Safeway
Medicated Shampoo Slednium Sulfide Dandruff Shampoo	up&up	Target	Target
Salon Shampoo (for Extra-Dry Hair)	Parnevu	Advantage Research Laboratories	Lynas Beauty Depot
Shea Butter Shampoo	Sofn'freen'pretty	M&M Products Company	Lynas Beauty Depot
Conditioning Shampoo	Luster's Pink Brand	Luster's Product	Lynas Beauty Depot
Coconut Oil Formula Conditioning Shampoo	Palmer's	E.T. Browne Drug Co.	Lynas Beauty Depot

Neutralizing Shampoo (With DL Panthenol)	Vitale	AFAM Concept	Lynas Beauty Depot
Extra Moisturizing Hand Wash	Dermasil/Rise International Group LLC	Rise International Group	99 Cent Only Stores
Moisturizing Shampoo with Panthenol (Placenta & Vitamin E)	La Bella	Newhall Laboratories, Inc.	99 Cent Only Stores
Despicable Me Hand Wash (tickled pink rose bonbon)	Delon Laboratories	Delon Laboratories	99 Cent Only Stores
Tingling Gro Shampoo with Flaking Control	Doo Gro	Nature's Protein	Sally Beauty Company
KeraCare Anti-Dandruff Moisturizing Shampoo	KeraCare	Avalon Industries, Inc.	Macy's
Dandruff Moisturizing Shampoo	Folicure	Alberto Culver USA	Sally Beauty Company
Mixed Berry Anti-Bacterial Foaming Hand Soap	Simple Pleasures	Tri-Coastal Design	Kohl's
Vanilla Rose Bubble Bath	Simple Pleasures	Paula Scaletta Licensed to Tri-Coastal Design	Kohl's
Berry burst shower gel	scentsations by bodysource	Made Especially for Kohl's Department Store	Kohl's
Lemon Hand Wash Gift Set	Brompton and Langley	Unlisted	Sears
French Lavender Hand and Body Wash Gift Set	Amelie's Garden	Unlisted	Sears
Moroccan oil Extra Volume Shampoo	Moroccan oil	Moroccan oil	Blooming Beauty
Julius Caesar Refreshing Citrus Scent Concentrated Shower Gel	Zirch Warrior Collection	TPR Holdings LLC	Marshalls
I love Vanilla & Ice Cream Bubble Bath and Shower Gel	I love . . .	I love cosmetics limited	Ross
Coconut Lime Hand soap	Pure Passion	Biolab International Inc.	Ross
Lalaloopsy Cotton Candy Bubble Bath	Lalaloopsy	Added Extras	Ross
Super Minty Soapy Suds Body wash + Bubbling Bath	Bliss	Bliss	Ross
Olive & Shea Moisturizing Shower Wash Vanilla Spice	Tree Hut	Naterra International	Ross
Organic Cleanse Deep Cleansing Shampoo with Oatmeal Protein	Design Essentials	McBride Research Laboratories	JC Penny
Moisturizing Shampoo for all hair types	Body Time	Body Time	Body Time
Lemon Kitchen Hand Soap	Trader Joe's	Trader Joe's	Trader Joe's
All Natural moisturizing Shower Gel Yuzu	ShiKai	ShiKai Products	Andronico's
2 in1 Shampoo and Conditioner	Toys R Us	Toys R Us	Babies R Us
Body Wash Ylang Ylang & ginger	Pharmaca	Pharmaca	Pharmaca
avocado oil moisturizing shower gel	Australian Organics	Kent Cosmetics	TJ Maxx
Lemon Balm White Musk Hand Wash	D&H Australia	Dickens & Hawthorne Australia	TJ Maxx

Eucalyptus Aloe Hand Soap	CST	CST	TJ Maxx
Honey B Crème Handwash	Scottish Fine Soaps	Scottish Fine Soaps Company	TJ Maxx
Enriched with Argan oil Restorative Shampoo	Beauty Products	Chic Cosmetic Ind.	TJ Maxx
White Nectarine & Pear Cleansing Hand Wash	Boutique	Grace Cole Co.	TJ Maxx
Lavender Conditioning Handwash	Brown & Harris England	Hot House Partnerships LTD	TJ Maxx
English Rose Moisturizing Hand Wash	A & S	Asquith & Somerset	TJ Maxx
Best Face Forward Daily Foaming Cleanser Passion fruit + Green Tea	Formula 10.0.6	Aspire Brands	Ultra
Triple Action Bath, Shower, & Hair Wash Revitalizing Rosemary Mint	c. Booth simple. Natural. Trusted.	Freeman Beauty Labs/ pH Beauty Labs	Ultra
Advanced Volume Shampoo with Expansion Technology	Nick Chavez	Perfect Plus	Ultra
Bubble Bath Calm One with lemon balm	Calm All	The Soap & Glory Cosmetics	Sephora
Lemon Basil Shea Butter Hand Soap	Michel Design Works	Michel Design Works	Bristol Farms
Philip B. Peppermint & Avocado Volumizing and Clarifying Shampoo	Phillip B.	Phillip B Inc.	Bloomingdale's
Lemon Verbena Hand Wash Gel	Accessory Zone	Accessory Zone	Sears
Mango Body Wash	Boots	The Boots Company	Target
Citrus Blush Shower Gel	Champneys	Boots Retail	Target
White Tea and Ginger Neutralizing Shampoo	Ampro/Pro Styl/ Neutra Foam	Ampro Industries	Lucky
Lychee Flower Hand And Body Wash	Mor	Mor	Nordstrom Rack
Zinc Shampoo	DHS	Person & Covey Inc.	hairenvy.com
Bubble Bath Sweet Water	RRYSpa	RRYSpa	Burlington coat factory
Skinny Girl Shower Gel Margarita	Skinny Girl	Lotta Luv	Burlington coat factory
Peppermint Bubble Bath	Elegant Home Design	Elegant Home Design	Burlington coat factory
Apothecary Lemon Verbena Bath and Shower Gel	Apothecary	International Design Associates	Burlington coat factory
French Lavender Cleansing Hand Wash	Baylis & Harding England	Baylis & Harding PLC	Burlington coat factory
American Crew Classic Daily Shampoo	American Crew	American Crew	Saks Fifth Avenue
Herb Hand Soap	Daiso	Daiso Industries	Daiso
Hair Plump Volumizing Shampoo	Big & Bold	Fisk Industries	Beauty Parlor
Blondes Lemon flower Shampoo	ARTEC	ARTec Systems Group	Beauty Parlor
Rejuvi Shower Cream	Rejuvi	Rejuvi Laboratory Inc.	Dermstore.com

The Revitalizer Body Wash (Cucumber + Grapefruit)	Portico	Portico Home + Spa	Dermstore.com
Colour Protecting Caviar Shampoo	Kelly Van Gogh	Kelly Van Gogh LLC	Dermstore.com
Walnut Body Scrub	Banzai Living Inc	Banzai Living Inc	Ichibankan
Clear Lemon & Mint Body Soap	Aroma Resort	PMAI	Ichibankan
Bath/Shower Gelee with Green Tea and Aloe	Dr. Michelle Copeland	Dr. Michelle Copeland Skin Care	Dermstore.com
Lavender Shower Gel with cucumber, arnica, and aloe vera	Elizabeth W san Francisco	E Wightman & Co	Dermstore.com

http://www.ceh.org/news-events/press-releases/content/lawsuit-launched-testing-finds-cancer-causing-chemical-in-100-shampoos-haircare-products/

There are some alternate herbs that will help enhance your hair grow and clean your hair without the harmful effects. Try Herbal options like:

Jojoba oil (is humectants that work great to reduce damage ends and promote healthier production.

Grapeseed oil added to your conditioner works well.

Aztec clay maybe found in either Bentonite clay or Red clay (detoxify your scalp),

Black soap (is one of the best natural cleansers),

Shea butter (adds moisture and softens the hair),

Rosemary and **mint** (stimulate hair growth by improving circulation, also great for hair dandruff. Don't forget the vinegar and the baking soda to help with any clarification or ph balance problems that may be apparent by how fast the hair dries when wet.

Vinegar (great for lowering the hair ph it is a great cleanser, antimicrobial, and antifungal agent)

Baking Soda (great neutralizing cleanser, odor eliminator helps reduce oil, and other product buildup)

TOOLS REQUIRED

Selecting the best styling tools for natural hair is very important. The use of a comb is not necessary for everyday styling of natural hair. Because natural curly hair may be coarse, the use of the wrong styling aid may cause more breakage or destruction to your hair. Black hair does not grow downward, it grows outward and draws close toward the scalp; therefore any combing the hair downward is not the most effective method for detangling. So I suggest using your finger to detangling, maybe a wide-tooth comb, or the Denman brush. Use of the Denman brush will help detangle the hair after a good shampooing and conditioning.

Try to use 4-8 clips in each section and detangle the hair very carefully. Make sure you avoid the clips with the metal because hair can get stuck, and you will notice more breakage.

A shower bonnet is great to help seal in the moisture, and also help the heat set in during your shower.

A good pair of sharp shears really helps keep the ends from splitting. Avoid any shears that you have used to cut paper, other fabrics or materials because the trimming will lead to more split ends or jagged edges. You can cut the hair wet or dry, but the best trimming is on completely dried-out stretched hair. I strongly recommend you go to a professional stylist for trimming of the hair if you have not been trained to clip your hair. Be aware that trimming and cutting your ends doesn't change the amount of growth that you will see, but it will help reduce tangling and breakage.

Now after washing the hair it is highly recommended to use a cotton towel or a 100% cotton t-shirt to reduce any friction or snagging of the hair that will cause additional breakage. The best clipping of the ends are done when the hair is wet, so dampen the ends using a spray bottle to spritz the hair as you clip the ends.

STYLING YOUR KINKS ON THE GO

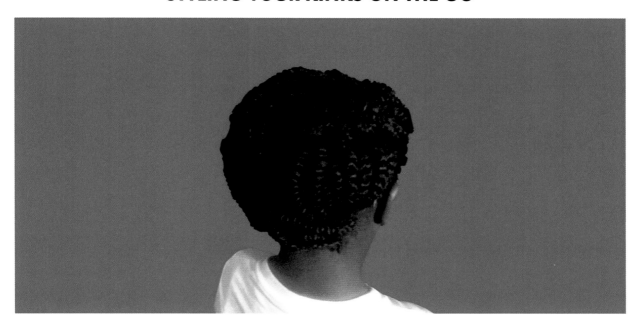

Natural hair can be convenient and quick to style. Typically wash-n-go is great for styling natural hair. Depending on your hair texture you may consider the use of a great styling crème or aid to achieve a nice, shiny curl. Curls will shrink and there are different anti-shrink formulas on the market to help stretch and elongate your curls. The biggest secret to the wash-n-go is to seal your hair with cold water after washing and conditioning your hair. The protein in the conditioners will help give your hair a nice appearance. Saturate the hair from the root to the ends with your favorite product, and make sure you avoid combing or any manipulations once the hair has been styled. Allow the hair to dry naturally or use a dryer. Once the hair is completely dried the curls will feel slightly crunchy and you will want to avoid touching the hair at this point until the hair has completely dried.

After you take out the braids or twist, it is important to not wash the hair right away but carefully detangle it to prevent gross breakage. Before shampooing I highly recommend you pre-poo, by preparing your hair with oil for extra protection. Conditioning is a critical step to help your hair after wearing any protective style for any length of time. The hair needs restoration treatment after any wearing any style that interferes with the cleansing process. Restoration care will help with environmental toxins removal, ph balance, moisture and hydration needed to keep the hair healthy. Again conditioners restore the protein and moisture balance.

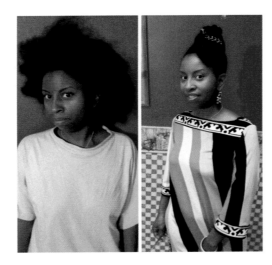

Pin up the hair nightly to keep the ends of your hair from getting damaged and it also will make a great style in the morning when you go to take your hair down. If you don't have pins or clips, you can always Bantu-knot the hair. You will notice a big difference in your wave pattern or curls. Bantu knots is just coiling the hair into a candy curl then taking the hair and rolling it around in a circular pattern to make the hair into one knot or a ball. Jada Pinkett-Smith wore Bantu knots in the movie *The Matrix*. Always place enough oil on your hands to help reduce the frizz and style the hair. Just remember to gently separate the hair from the root with your hands by splitting the hair to create more curls, and avoid the comb for the best control styles that last the entire day.

Curl activator is great for a wet look and it also helps low porous hair by adding the humectants to help keep the hair from drying. Hair will appear oily, shiny, and moist when you use the curl activator. You will not want to use it all the time because it can cause skin breakouts. I always seal my hair with gel after applying any activator and you should let the style and moisture set by the use of the dryer.

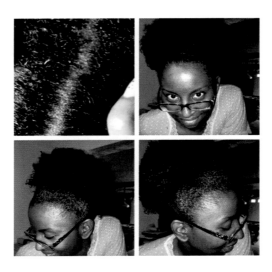

WEATHER PROOF YOUR HAIR

During seasonal changes the hair requires different types of protection. The hair needs to be protected from the UV rays of the sun, ice-cold weather, and wind. I did not include the rain because a little rain never hurts my hair, but a lot of women use extra precaution for the rain and they are not as concerned when it comes to the hot sun or the extreme cold weather. I notice in Florida the salt water and the sun causes my hair to be a little thirstier. Funny right? The hair can become thirsty in Sunny Florida and more hydration and moisture balance are required. Braids are great for the South, East coast and West coast because of the humidity. Styling of natural hair maybe a challenge because of frizzing of the hair occurs in the southern regions. Today to avoid the harmful effects of the sun rays, some hair care products are introducing the UV protection and the SPF. But to be very honest, SPF protection is really limited after so many hours of exposure, and I really am not sure how effective the blockers are. I don't know if it is worth the investment to get a product that has the SPF included because after you hit the water all protection is spilled in the water not in your hair. I highly recommend large sun hats, swim caps, nice braids, and remember it is important to condition the hair prior to styling or braiding.

Now understand Chemistry 101 any product that is on your hair while you go swimming in chlorinated water will have an impact and you must use corrective shampoos or conditioners to wash out the chlorine. I generally use condition on my hair prior to swimming. I have also saturate my hair with mineral oil; although I do not recommend mineral oil , but it works well to seal my hair prior to taking the swim. Leave-in conditioners are not typical heavy enough to prevent the hair from damage from the sun and the chlorine. Prior to any good swim you must read your labels again, if the product contains lots of preservatives you will need to avoid it during you swim. I like to apply conditioner to my hair then saturate my hair with mineral oil. I braid the hair down to protect my ends. Now if I don't have time to wash my hair or care for my hair after the swim, I wear a plastic cap during my swim. Be aware that some of your hair will be exposed to the chlorine, so I generally give my hair a nice washing after any swim. If your hair is braided during the swim it is vital that you wash, condition and rinse the hair after the swim because your hair will suffer great damage after the prolonged exposure to the water. Living in the tropics is nice, but our hair is often affected by our climate, and we must educate ourselves on how to care for the hair during the extreme hot weather.

I really don't know much about the cold and ice, but it seems like my tropical hair loves the opportunity to get out of the extreme weather like hot climates and adapts nicely to cold climates. I notice less damage and hair growth from the extremely weather. I am not sure if it is because I prepare myself for the cold and cover my head when I go out. In the cold weather it is important to cover the hair when you go out, but be careful to not cover the hair too much because the scalp needs to breath and the cotton caps may cause friction and breakage if worn for extended length of time. Do not forget to oil your hair a little more in the cold weather because your hair generally dries out and requires a nice oil and moisture balance. Hydration is another story. Hydration is the water balance; hair becomes very thirsty and slightly dehydrated during the extreme cold weather. Flaking occur, but oil will not solve that problem, the hair needs a little water, which is hydrogen and oxygen to survive. This is why I say covering the head for too long is never good.

Protective styling is great for the prevention of breakage. Shoulder length hair has a tendency to rub against the fibers in your clothes and causes the ends to become frail and breakage occurs. If you have short hair, the hair is not as prone to the same breakage so it is recommended to try up styles, buns, ponytails, braids, and French rolls. If you work in large corporations, it is recommended to do more protective styling than allowing your hair to go below the shoulder. Hair below the shoulder is not as clean and may create a large dry cleaning bills, because of the oils on the end hitting against your clothes. Wearing your hair down depends on the fabric you are wearing. Try silk clothing or go sleeveless when you want to wear your hair down to prevent breakage. Hair pins, hair combs, clips may or may not be a great options for pin ups. Satin ponytail holders and no break ponytails really work well. I love the comb around my crown to give my short ponytail the appearance of a full thick pony tail. Bands and other methods can easily be used to keep the friction to a minimum.

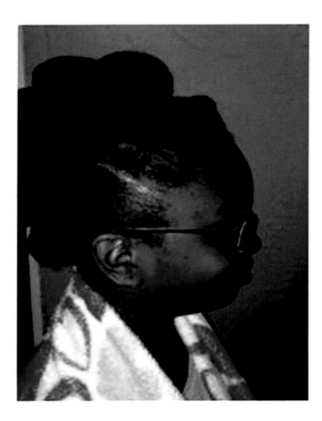

Braids, twists, flat twists, shingles, braid out, Bantu knots, coiling, or coil outs are other great styles for natural hair. These styles are easy to do and generally styling them requires little to no time to style without the use of chemicals. Natural hair does not require a comb! The nice thing about the natural hair is that it really has great staying power; if you styled it yesterday, the next day the hair should be a simple fluff out with your fingers. Wearing a scarf for protection will keep your hair intact, I highly recommend the satin bonnet or wrap. Scarves help prevent breakage and it also prevents your hair from drying out. Honestly the longer your hair, the easier it is for you to do more protective styles. When twisting or styling your hair, which requires the comb for parting, try the end of a rattail comb to make the parting much easier. Also, try not to worry so much about the part being perfect. Natural hair is thick and normally not perfect. So the desire to make natural hair look perfect really is not reasonable. Research different styling tips to prevent you from getting too bored with the same old style. Alternate your hair accessories and try different accessories like pearls, flowers of different kinds and sizes, stylish hair pins, buttons, and other unique styles. Any accessory added to your high up bun will make your style look unique and add an extra pizzazz.

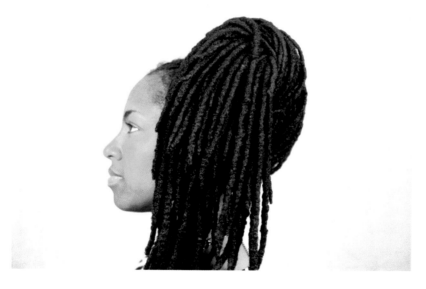

You can roll natural hair at night and protect the hair with a satin bonnet. In the morning when styling it, forget the comb; just use your hands to detangle or style your hair. Make sure to use the oil on your hands to help you separate the hair easier. The oil will help add more shine and reduce the frizz. Spread each section of hair apart gently. Do not over style the hair and keep pulling on the hair because you will cause the hair to appear frizzy, and the extra manipulations will make the hair look uneven and dull.

Straw set and other commercial rolling techniques can be use to give yourself a nice classy curl. Curl Formers give a beautiful candy curl. Any curl styling can be obtained by proper handling of the hair or by a professional stylist that has experience with caring for natural hair. Some curls require a little styling gel or crème for a great hold. Oil is required for any of the curls to add a little sheen to the hair. Heat is also great to seal in the shine and help the style last a little longer. If you are not fond of heat, I recommend you roll the hair and let it set over night to get the optimal curly look. But be aware that unprocessed hair does not require a comb; if you do comb the hair be aware that the hair will frizz, and the defined curl pattern will be compromised. Explore all different types of commercial curling products to find the best curling aides that matches you hair styling needs.

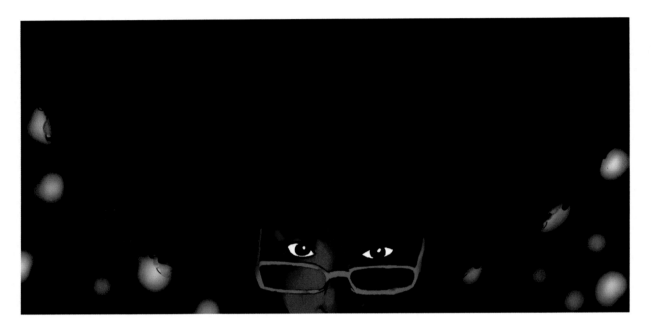

The Bantu knot seems to be one of the most popular styles for curly kinks, because it stretches the hair and gives it beautiful volume. It is a great protective style and it can be done easily every night by simple 2 strand twists or on untwisted hair. All you need to do is create a round ball and wrap the hair in circular motions around the ball until the ends get trapped or sealed into the ball. I call this technique 'the Naturals wrap'. If you ever want to show your hair length without the heat the Bantu knots is the way to go. You can also dry the hair and twist, or Bantu knot the hair to give you full volume. Try to separate the hair very carefully so the hair styling remains even and controlled. It also helps reduce the frizz. Make sure after you unravel the knot you carefully style, avoiding combing or too much pulling, because you will get frizz and the definition in the style will not look as appealing.

Frizz can be caused by the atmosphere, improper care, and poor handling of the hair, and can easily be resolved with the use of cold water, moisturizer, and less manipulation. Always start with freshly washed hair, condition, and then apply your product. Try not to comb or touch your hair once the hair is fully saturated and ready to go. Conditioned hair frizzes less. The hair is clean, shiny, and requires little to no attention. Let the hair air dry and avoid any heat at this point. If you go back and touch the hair you will notice the frizz will begin. There is a campaign to discourage others from touching natural hair because natural hair does not like to be touched. It is very sensitive!

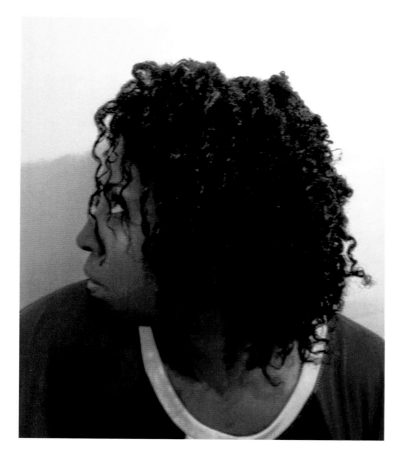

If you really don't like the shrunken look you can try banding methods to help the hair stretch as it dries. I have used the Aluminum foil to band my hair by wrapping the hair into small sections after I apply product to avoid the dreadfully short look. After washing the hair simply condition and detangle. Part the hair into 4 small equal sections. Use a light moisturizing oil then ponytail the hair into about 4 ponytails. Some bloggers suggest banding with the no elastic ponytail holders in multiple parts along the length of your hair and allowing it to dry completely without the use of heat. This method is real helpful and the hair is stretched nicely.

Cornrows are the easiest and most customary look. It is not surprising that some people have not mastered the technique of how to cornrow or braid from the scalp in a downward pattern. There is no easy written tutorial on how to braid. Practice taking one piece of hair and crossing it over each strand of hair in a pattern a few times and hopeful you will eventually learn or develop how to braid you hair. You can do as little as 4 and increase the cornrows as you feel comfortable. Hair does not have to be long for the cornrow. You can cornrow hair that is barely one inch and create a nice look. The benefit of the cornrow on short hair is it stretches the hair and helps with growth, as long as you are not applying too much tension.

Fish tail braids are a new European surprise that has been spread and shared within the United States.

Some regions have large contests to determine the best fish tail style. You can give each braid a fuller look by lightly pulling the ends out evenly as you are braiding down. For this style, your hair will have to be long, stretched out, and it may require a little extension to give you a more full detailed look. This style is great for protection and growth.

I will not even begin to complicate your life by trying to provide a written instructional on this technique; my suggestion is to go to YouTube and find a great tutorial and watch it a few times and try it. I am sure once you have mastered this technique your friends and family will be asking for your help with this type of braid. This style looks best on straighten hair; it is really too complicated and does not look very neat on curly or short hair.

Try the Bow tie. As your hair gets longer you can try different tying techs that are unique and different from the rest. Take two sections and tie the hair in a knot; then wrap the hair around in your fingers and make two loops and bow tie them together. The hair has to be very long, or you may need to add some synthetic hair to make the look full and voluminous. You can get creative and tie 3 or more knots going down the center to create a Mohawk look. Don't forget to accessorize to give your hair a unique artistic appeal for special occasions.

Natural hair can easily be straighten with the use of a flat iron or curling iron, but the use of heat protection will be necessary to prevent the harmful drying effects of any heat source. I love my ion ceramic heating tool because it adds some extra protection to the hair. My flat iron prevents my hair from burning. The ion heating tools (like the tourmaline) causes negative charges, which help the hair lock in the moisture to enhance the hydration and prevent the frizz. The ceramic actually allows a seal to form around the hair and coats the hair to protect the hair. Ceramic material really heat from the inner cuticle to the cortex. Be aware that the best heating tools are expensive, but are well worth the investment. Also, look for heating tools with temperature adjustments. They all go up to about 450 degrees but this can add great injury to your hair. After you finished using the heating tool, make sure you keep your equipment clean because any burned oil will cause smoking and burning of your hair if not removed. I would suggest, like anything else, for you to do your research when paying for very expensive hair styling equipment and see other product reviews; because what works for some people may not work well for you.

Because hair styles becomes a challenge when you work for a large corporation or in the US armed forces, or when you work out daily, I want to take a moment to help you understand your options and resources. I understand there are more limitations on the styles you can wear because of company policies, procedures, company standards, or etiquette. Short neat boy cuts work well, but the makeup is a must. Try pinup styles that are neatly groomed. Ponytail may or may not be appropriate depending on the length of the hair. Hair really needs to be very clean and tidy. Try hair extension for more options. Weaves and wigs are also great when you are working under strict standards. But, you must not forget to take care of your own natural hair. Weekly washing and deep conditioning are required.

Salon styling with guidance works well for the everyday women and the everyday look. I know that the book has been geared toward avoiding chemicals and loving your unprocessed hair, but I do not want anyone to be discouraged. Some women love the European or straight look and there is nothing wrong with that. Wearing natural or unprocessed hair may provide a lot of options, and straightened hair is definitely one of them. The nice thing about natural straight hair is that it may give you a much fuller, healthier look and there are much more options for styling. Some people wear their natural hair and you would never even think it was natural. I have just gotten so accustomed to my curls and the low maintenance of wash and go. I have not really been interested in straightening. I will tell you if you straighten natural hair with a hot comb or flat iron at a high temperature or running heat about 3 times in a row, you will notice the curl pattern will change. The curls tend to revert and you will find the ends of your hair to be straight all the time. If you flat iron your hair you will need to wear heat protection. This will help you avoid the damage from the heat. Honey and molasses works really well to help seal your hair and help with humidity. These heat protection products work really well, but if you do not have any heat protection product the Aloe Vera gel will help protect the hair.

If you are not very creative with your styling just try a wig, but make sure your hair is braided under the wig; your hair care is still very important so when you get home the wig needs to come off. If you are working out, maybe try a scarf, sweatband, ponytail style, wrap, pin up, or any style that will keep your hair up and off your neck or face. The goal when you are working out is sweat and there are unique head gear. Protective cotton head device can be worn to keep your hair from getting wet.

Styles that work great for women who work out are very dependent on your creativity. Vinegar helps the hair stay clean and fresh if you are wearing any style for any length of time. I say use vinegar because sweating and wet hair can cause to stimulates for any length of time can cause mold and other bacteria to grow easily. Women who wear their hair up in a ponytail should always check your scalp and keep it clean and fresh at all times. Twist-up styles works well for women that work out and the use of a sweatband will help keep the sweat from causing the frizz.

High and low buns work nicely for weather protective styling and for a nice night out on the town. Hair needs to be detangled, washed, and clean for better styling. Brush all hair in an upward motion and put the ponytail toward the center of your head. If you hair is not long enough to give that full appearance I recommend khaki synthetic hair to wrap around the ponytail. Once the hair is neatly in place I advise you to apply something to the ends to help the hair stay in place, I like gels or pomades, and they work well for me all day. After the hair has been styled and put into place I recommend you apply your scarf for about 20 minutes to seal the style and give you a nice controlled look and people will think you spent hours straighten your hair to get it up in the bun. For a night out on the town or the holiday parties add some sparking beads or an old necklace for the wraparound to accessorize the hairstyle.

Don't assume all straight hair is created equally. Some straight hair is chemically relaxed, a weave, or just flat ironed hair. It really is not complicated to achieve the straight look. I highly recommend shampooing and using deep conditioner. Next apply some clear leave in conditioner or protein. Then apply a good moisturizing sealant to protect the hair from heat damage. There are products on the market to help prepare the hair for the heat. I have worked with my own homemade hair stretching formulas inspired by Etae caramelizing treatment, which adds some essential vitamins like potassium, protein, oil, and molasses. After the hair has been prepped for the styling you need to detangle completely. Blow-dry and use some heat protection to prevent any hair loss. After the hair is completely dry simply go over the hair with the flat iron, try to avoid going through the hair with the heating appliance more than 2 times. Avoiding any prolong exposures of the heat to the hair with prevent permanent damage to the hair. The ion and the ceramic plates help seal the hair and create some extra protection. Heat damage is significantly reduced by the use of the correct flat iron. There are some steam ceramic ion flat irons that do not dry the hair, but the hair has to be detangled before applying the steam dryer flat iron. Precaution the temp setting at 450 degree and with the steam temperature can be much higher than traditional heat stylers.Make sure you use the devices properly and don't get too stuck on making the hair bone straight as though you were born with straight hair. Be yourself and wear the hair that you were born with proudly. Take care of your hair and make sure you wrap the hair and use you silk/satin scarf. Now if the hair smells burn it maybe your warning that your hair may have gotten burnt. To camouflage the burnt smell you may want to get your favorite perfume spray in the palm of your hands, rub them together, then clap the hands together, and rub the dry palm of your hands through your dry hair. Your hair will freshen up and you can also spray your scarf, but make sure it is dry before reapplying it to your hair.

I do not recommend Keratin treatments and Brazilian blow-outs. The extra chemicals change the pH and the structure of your hair. They may potentially cause more protein build up to your hair, which may lead to more breakage. If you do not understand chemicals I want to encourage you not to try any chemicals that will potentially put your hair at risk of damage or breakage.

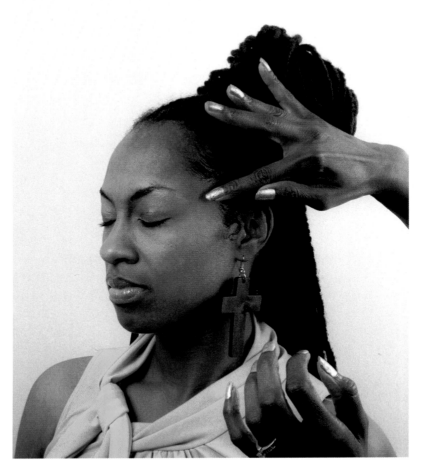

DREAD HAIR CARE

Dreading the hair makes it easy for styling. Using a comb method and twisting the hair makes a great style that requires little to no hair care. I recommend you find a good locktician to start your dreads. Coiling method is not a quick start, but once the hair is completely coiled you will not have to worry much about daily hair styling, but this style is not a budget balancing style. You have to be prepared to go to the salon regularly for the edges of the hair to be nice. Massaging the scalp is an important way to stimulate growth for dreaded hair. I recommend nightly massages to help with the stimulation of the scalp and aid in relaxation. Also I recommend covering the hair with a silk scarf at night to avoid breakage and damage caused by dryness, and lent build up in the dreads. I also recommend with dread hair you avoid too much tension. Any tight styling even the ponytail can potentiate hair loss around the edges. Please don't forget the basics of all hair care and keep the scalp clean and dry. Clean the scalp and try a little witch hazel between shampooing to relief itching. Shampooing regularly remains very important when you wear locs. Layering the scalp with oil is not recommended, and the use of thick heavy products build up over time, like waxing, is not recommended. If wax is used, I recommend a nice clarifying cleanser, vinegar, or try a baking soda mix, but be careful about hair care products stripping the hair and remove oil from the hair. I generally use vinegar to remove product build up and clarify the hair. For itching, I may use baking soda to help control the ph imbalance and neutralize the hair's ph. Keep in mind that locs may have a white film in the scalp that may not be easily removed; if you over clarify the scalp this film will disappear, but you may strip the natural oils produced in the scalp and you will notice more flaking or dandruff from the stripping of your natural oils. Try to wash the hair regularly to avoid excessive build up and to keep the dreaded hair clean and refreshed.

NATURAL HAIR CARE FOR KIDS

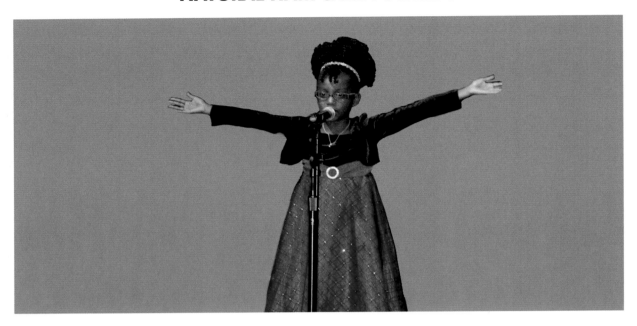

Remember the motto, "Keep it so simple when caring for your child's hair." Simple hair care is essential although children's hair is more resistant, and we must be very gentle and careful with their hair. Try to avoid the use of multiple products. Do a simple weekly cleaning using a mild cleanser. It is a good idea to use a combination of oils to avoid products mixing because children have different hair chemistry than adults. Less is best when it comes to the child. Less manipulation, less pulling of the scalp, less oiling, and less styling is the greatest guides for children hair care. When using oils we highly recommend you use a satin scarf at night to help with the oil retention and reduce friction. Cotton t-shirts work well for drying hair also. Pay close attention to their scalp daily because pathogens or bacteria invade the scalp quickly and require quick and immediate attention. The use of vinegar is a great cleanser for children because it will reduce any pathogens that cause scalp infections or irritations. You also want to consider a mild, gentle shampoo. Stick with what works and try to avoid product swapping and the use of new products on the market. Remember a change in hormones for girls begin around the age of 12, hair will become very different in texture and may not be conducive to some products. You may have change your product and consider deep conditioning with a combination of oil treatments to prevent hormonal hair loss. Encourage all children to eat properly, drink plenty of water and try a daily vitamin supplement to improve their hair growth. Sometimes a professional stylist may help improve the overall quality of the hair and to help detangle the hair. Detangling is very important, and I advise the youth to try sectioning the hair off into big braids and then shampooing the hair to prevent too much tangling. This method allows you to cleanse the scalp better. I have many techniques I use for my daughter's hair and she loves the results, and I love the shortcuts because it easy for me to wash and care for. I warn you that young hair requires a lot more attention to the fine details. Styling takes much longer. Being patient and using the styling session as an opportunity to bond will help the little princess feel like she is worth your time and energy. After completing the styling, make sure you tell her how beautiful she is and get her honest opinion about how she feels. Children and young hair care needs to remain simple.

I strongly suggest testing your products before applying any product to your child's hair. I've learned through experience because my daughter has so many food and environmental allergies, and she is at great risk for losing her hair in the future. My uncle developed large boils in his hair and on his skin. He went to several doctors to determine what the cause of the lesions was. The lesions become worse, and caused significant hair loss. He had no idea and had nowhere to turn when it came to treatment of these grossly annoying lesions. Finally, after a series of test and a visit to the dermatologist they determined he had a gluten and wheat allergy. Gluten allergies are crucial allergy, and it is very important to discover it at birth. However, my uncle went on a strict modified diet which and changed the course of his life forever. My daughter also tested positive for soy, wheat, peanut, gluten, and tested positive for celiac disease. I only noticed her abdominal distention, she suffered from severe excruciating abdominal pain after she ate certain foods. Gluten is a binder and we know more about the binding effects causes constipation and poor digestion of her meals. Now if we had not corrected her diet and meal plan she would have been at risk for long-term effects of the allergy. The Interesting fact is that the gastroenterology doctor said we couldn't starve this child and not allow her to eat the food. We must give her the Lactulose to remove the binding effects to her body. Now do you see the problem? My daughter is at risk as she gets older for hair loss. She has a beautiful head of 12 more inches of hair. She is very quick to say to me, "Wash my hair". Now I have not determined the best hair care for her hair, because my hair is not the same as her hair. The secret for her hair is, after I wash her hair we don't apply much oil. I apply a little coconut oil once a week, and that is it. Her scalp is trained that way, and she is happy without all the product buildup. Her hair grows at least 6 inches per year. Her hair length could be a lot longer if she would focus on her diet, drink more water, scalp massage, and some deep conditioners.

My point in telling you about my daughter is to convey that we all have something unique and different about our hair, and it is important to determine what uniquely works best. First of all, stop thinking that just because your child has long pretty locks and a beautiful shine, her hair is always going to be like that way. You must understand allergies, medical conditions, and hormones will have a large effect on your Child's hair. Stop treating your child's hair the way you treat your hair. Wash the hair, keep a clean scalp, avoid short cuts, and start giving your child a supplement will help grow the hair. Now be forewarned, a lot of vitamins may contain something your child may be allergic to. I suggest good diet, preventive actions and healthy living will help your child with the hair care. I know this may sound ridiculous, but a little Jell-O goes a long way with any hair growth. Jell-O contains protein, and it helps with the elasticity of the hair. Avoid any petroleum to the scalp and try a sealant and protection that will not cause death to the ends of your hair; focus on something that will cause all living cells to be nurtured. Coconut, honey, hair milk, and leave in conditioners will change your child's hair significantly. I suggest less tension to the scalp (pulling and tight braids); loose braids, flat twists, and two strand twists works well for the young girls. Try to avoid heat if possible unless their hair is high porous hair that easily develops a fungus. Fungus is an awful invasion of the wet scalp. All kinds of bacteria and fungus grow in the scalp. Once fungus develops you must wash properly, use an antifungal agent and then dry only the high porous hair from the scalp to the ends. High porous hair holds onto the water and does not dry rapidly. High porous hair requires more hair care and attention only a few times a week which allows the scalp to breath, but try not to braid the hair in a tight, tiny braid unless your plan is to wash it with the braids in and do not skip the complete drying process along with a little oil. Now can your child wear the Afro puffs all day? Let's be realistic, yes, but the weather will determine if the hair will like being unprotected. Protective styling is best for all kids. I love braids, plaits, and twists hair for kid's hair styling. Regarding un-protective hair styling, it may be ok in the summer time, when there is no wind in the air. I hate to tell you this, but you must teach your children not to touch the hair once it has been styled, and also make sure others know that the hands will make the hair frizzy and make it look a hot mess. Regarding un-protective styling, you can try less hand manipulation, no combing, enough oil, and a thick leave in conditioner or a good hair care product. But for unprotected hair you will have to wash the hair after two days, because the hair will have all kinds of atmospheric particles that will attach itself to the hair. An example is pollen may build up with the conditioners in the hair the child's hair will look like it has not been washed.

As a reminder, I recommend twist, big braiding, ponytails, Bantu knots, flat twist, and extensions if they are going to wear the braid for any length of time or for swimming. Refer to the shampooing section of this guide to understand how to protect your hair for swimming.

MEN'S HAIR CARE

Now washing of the men's hair is a little simple, in that they can wash their hair weekly. I advise them to co-wash or wash the hair with conditioner. Afro-American men who wear the hair in a low cut have to focus on scalp care. Avoid the use of dull razors or razors close to the scalp because it may cause scar tissue nodules or keloids. Keloids are large bumps, growth, or scar tissue formation. Keloids can be itchy, painful, and are uneven texturing to your scalp. If you have this problem, try not to let it grow too big; seek the advice of a dermatologist for help with keloid or any other abnormal scalp issues. They normally recommend steroid treatment or removal to help reduce the undesirable appearance. Keloids are very common in Afro-American men, and must be treated with care. Crew cuts are nice and the military loves to skin the hair off the face and the scalp, but it causes irreversible damage and an ungodly appearance to the Afro-American man.

Also, make sure you always take extra precautions to avoid the infections of the scalp. A little oil goes a long way. Try Tea Tree oil to help improve the scalp and reduce any potential risk. I suggest using a nice clean hairbrush. Keep the hair simple; never use too much product; and make sure you always keep the scalp clean and dry.

Men who wear their hair long require a little more attention. I suggest finding a nice salon that can meet your needs because good hair care is imperative. For most men hair growth may not be a big deal since the wearing of long hair remains a restriction in some workplaces. Also remember that men's hair growth is not restricted by the hormonal changes like the hair growth in women.

Men should abide by corporation regulatory guidelines when wearing long hair. Even today with the Samson mentality, men have to be mindful of company's standards about the wearing of long hair. Personally, I find it attractive to see a man with long, clean, trimmed, and tapered around the edges hair. Wearing of suits, ties and dress shirts while wearing long hair is not very tidy, because hair below the neckline causes 'ring around the collar'. To maintain a professional appearance your clothes may have to be dry cleaned more often. For the companies you choose to work for, make sure all dreads are within the guideline of the dress code.

Just use my simple hair care plan for men's hair care and growth. I recommend men keep their hair care simple. Dilute your shampoos with water and try co-washing instead of daily cleaning. Try avoiding close shaving of the scalp with the razors to prevent scarring. Cutting twice a week instead of cutting daily will help prevent any infections from the razors. Keep your hair clean, tapered, and seek medical attention for any keloids.

SIMPLE HAIR CARE PLAN

Drink plenty of water
- Set a realistic goal of _____(1000 cc) cups per days.
- Take hair vitamins that include Biotin, Collagen, Vitamin B, Fe/ Iron.

Eat a healthy well balanced meal.
- Add protein, fiber, vegetable, and fruits.

Exercise
- Set goal _____times per week.
- Try Yoga or the Inversion method.

Massage your scalp
- Try organic oil_____.

Shampoo and cleanse
- Pre-poo_____ times per week.
- Condition or co-wash_____ times a week.

Try less manipulating styles
- Change style every _____2-3 days.
- Avoid the heat.
- Avoid combing.
- Detangle regularly.

Nubia's Favorite YouTube Natural Hair Vloggers:

NATURAL NUBIAN

Natural85
Curly Nikki
Nappturality
Taren Guy
Beautiful Brown Baby
Kinky Curly Coily
Pretty Dimples
Mahogany Curls
Rochelle-Black Onyx77
Kimmy Kim 416

Links: www.naptural85.com/, www.curlynikki.com/, www.nappturality.com/ , www.taren916.com/, www.beautifulbrwnbabydol.com/, www. kinkycurlycoilyme.com, www.prettydimples.com/, www.mahoganycurlsofficial.com, www.mahoganycurlsofficial.com, www.alikaynaturals.com, www.kimmykim416.com/

Some other vloggers include: MyNaturalSistas, Iknowlee, NaturalHairRules, Alicia James, Naturally Curly, Luvbeinnatural, Chary Jay, Natural Chica, Chime Edwards—Hair Crush, Janelle Stewart, The Natural Sistas, Simplyounique ,The Chic Natural, Bronze Goddess 01, LovelyAnneka, Jouelzy, Classcie, KG Lifestyle, Razorempress, and Long Hair Don't Care.

CONCLUSION

Design your own hair care plan when going natural. Stick with the same hair care routine, be patient, and try some great protective styling tips, by your favorite YouTube Vloggers to give your natural hair a variety of styles. I suggest when selecting a YouTube video you try to select someone whose hair that is similar to your hair type. If you are non-African American descent, try more organic, natural hair care solutions to improve the appearance of your hair. Exercising regularly helps in the development of healthy hair. After you learn your hair and what works best for your hair share your journey with your friends so they can feel more comfortable with their hair care regimen.

Stop chemically relaxing your hair or using alkaline products that destroy your hair's molecular structure. Opting to do the big chop will allow the hair to grow out healthier. Wearing protective styles will help you gain hair length, so the big chop is not necessary to go natural. I recommend protective styling be worn anywhere from 6 months to one year. The goal is only to see curly ends. Eat right, exercise, drink plenty of water, and try a vitamin supplement. Once you have found the correct balance from the inside you will be able to focus on a healthy hair care regimen. Try different natural oils and hair care products that are organic. Cold water after washing and less manipulation will help reduce the frizz. Never be afraid to apply a little oil no matter what type hair you have. Focus on the appearance of your scalp versus the appearance of the hair, because your unhealthy scalp will shed more. I recommend avoiding the hair trauma of tangling your hair when washing your hair. Use a nice gentle cleaning method, avoidance of the harsh shampoos and four section cleansing will help cleanse your scalp. Because the ends never get sebum or our natural oil, the applications of oil will help seal the ends and help cleanse dirt. Co wash, pre-poo, or whatever other technique depends on whatever works best for you. Cleanse your hair using non-chemical preserved shampoos; try black soap, vinegar, or baking soda. Any avoidance to all manmade and harsh chemicals will help improve your hair transform. Avoid all Sulfates, Paraben, Cocamide, Alcohol, and any chemical that you just can't pronounce.

Then do your research. Never be the first to try something you don't know about. If you understand chemicals and products, you will learn what may cause damage to your hair.

Have fun exploring some styling tips with our favorite YouTube celebrities and bloggers. Keep a photo journal to know how much you have accomplished and share your journey to a happy, healthy head of hair. If you have any medical conditions, please make sure, you are complying with your doctor's recommendations and focus on prevention to avoid the lifelong use of medications that may cause hair loss. Hope you enjoy Nubia's Guide To Going Natural. This book teaches you the scientific facts about going natural. There is something it in it for everyone. Men's hair care, kid hair care, and the everyday hair care will find something of great value to help them with their hair care and everyday maintenance of going natural. Try to unleash your curls and share this book with a friend.

GLOSSARY

DEA – is a derivative of Cocamide DEA or Lauramide DEA or Monoetholamine DEA and it can effect brain development.

Paraben interferes with your endocrine system and is found commonly in soap and shampoos.

The key to avoid any chemicals 1.4 Dioxane the organic consumers urge us to avoid products ending with "eth" like Laureth, Oleth, Certerareth, or and words ending in "oxynol" or "pol"

Saw palmetto blocks the testosterone to DHT-Dihydrotestosterone with cause's permanent alopecia. MSM is another supplement that helps improves hair growth by increasing the Anagen phase of hair growth

Burdock—is a plant found in China and Europe that is commonly used to purify your blood, it can be used to treat cancer, improve your digestive system, and acne, and other skin disorders. It contains Carbohydrates, volatile oils, plant sterols, tannins, and fatty acids.[2]

Sulfates—are mineral salts that contain Sulfur. It is used as a chemical preservative and can cause gastro disorders and asthma attacks. It is produced from decayed plants, animals, and some industrial processes. It is very harmful to our bodies. www.dhs.wisonsin.gov

Sulfur – is one of the most commonly found chemical elements, it is water soluble and can be burned to form a gas. It is an essential element for life. It is great for cell development and hair growth in its purest unaltered form. This is not to be confused with Sulfate or sulfites

Palmitic—is a waxy crystalline saturated acid $C16H32O2$ in the form of glycerin and form in most fatty acids and essential oils. www.Merriam-webster.com

Lauric Acid—is a medium chain fatty acid, commonly found in coconut oil. It converts different chemicals or minerals and exhibits antiviral, antiprotozoa, and antimicrobial properties. www. Natural news.com

EPA—Eicosapentaenoic acid—is another form of Omega 3 unsaturated fatty acids, commonly found in fish oil and is healthy for ingestion. www.supplementnews.org/ EPA

DHA—Docosahexaenoix—another form of the Omega3 fatty acid it is essential in brain development for the infants and other neurological disorders like ADHA—Attention Deficit Hyperactivity, Depression and other medical problems unassociated with the brain like Lupus and more. DHA can be found in cold water fatty fish and in seaweed. It is not harmful for ingestion or topic use. www.Umm.edu

Methylchloroisothiazolinone-is a preservative with antibacterial and antifungal effects. It works well with gram negative and positive bacteria. This is a substitute of parabens and it can cause allergic reactions and is a preservative or irritant. It reserves the products on the shelf to prevent spoiling or bacteria growth.

Ammonium chloride—is inorganic mechanically engineered water soluble salt, this is used to make the shampoos thicker.

Zeaxantin—one of the most common caroteneoid alcohols found in nature. Best source found in green leaves and is great for the eyes and health. www.aoa.org

Beta-carotene alpha carotene Lutein linoleic, oleic, and stearic, palmitic, Mystristic, and lauric mega 3, Omega 6, ALA or apha-linolenic acid which converts into the EPA – Eicosapentaenoic acid and DHA—docosahexaenoix acid

Mystristic—a fatty acid of lipid.

INDEX

WEBSITE RESOURCES

www.Altmedicine. about.com;

[1] www.stylecraze.com/?s=Vitamin+c; Source www.Stylecraze.com/articles/amazing-benefits—of-vitamin-c-for-skin-hair-and-health/;

[2] www.Umm.edu/health/medical/ altmed/herb/burdock;

[3] www.blackgirllonghair.com/2013/02/how-to-use-olive-oil-on-natural-hair/;

[5] www.Peppermintoilforhair.com;

[6] www.Naturallycurly.com/curlereading/kinky-hair-type-4a/5-ways-to-use-aloe-vera-gel/; www.longlocks.com; http://site.thegreenlifeonline.org/2012/04/30/finding-a-safe-shampoo-and-what-ingredients-to-avoid/;

www.Naturallycurly.com/curleading/kinky-hair-type-4a/5-ways-to-use-aloe-vera-gel/;

[7] www.Peppermintoilforhair.com; www.Nenonatural.com;

[8] www.Supergrowlasers.com/vitamins-to-help-growth.php;

[9] www.truehairgrowth.com;

[11] www.Med-health.net/Castor-Oil-For-Hair.html;

[12] www.livestrong.com/article/138885-how-to-use-stinging-nettle-hair—loss/#page=1; http://www.iheartmyhair.com/back-basics-must-styling-tools-curls-coils-kinks/;

[13] www.Livestrong.com/sscat/vitamins-supplements/; www.Nenonatural.com

[14] www.Sawpalmettohairlossreviews.com;

[15] www.Judymcfarland.com/skin.shtml;

[16] http://www.mayoclinic.org/drugs-supplements/flaxseed-and-flaxseed-oil/background/hrb-20059416-

[17] http://moroccanoilreviews.net;

[18] www.Blackgirllonghair by cipriana Nov 28, 2011;

[20] www.Livestrong.com/sscat/vitamins-supplements/;

www.livestrong.com/article/138885-how-to-use-stinging-nettle-hair—loss/#page=1;

[21] www.urbanbushbabes.com;

[25] www.livestrong.com/article/444501-does-vitamin-a-cause-hair-loss/#page=6;

[27] www.Blackgirllonghair by cipriana Nov 28, 2011;

[28] www.wheatgermbenefits.com/wheat-germ-oil/;

[29] www.Oilsofaloha.com/Kukui-skin-and Hair Care/; www.enslow.com;

www.mountainroseherbs.com/products/Kukui-nut-oil/profile ; www.Merriam-webster.com; www.supplementnews.org/ EPA; www.Umm.edu ; www.aoa.org; www.Natural news.com; www.dhs.wisonsin.gov

BOOK REFERENCES

Super Natural Home by Beth Greer(Podale 2009)

Hair Care Millionaire by Edwin Brit Wyckoff (Enslow2011)

Madame CJ Walker, by Patricia Fredrick McKissack

The Hundred –Year—How to Protect Yourself from the Chemicals That Are Destroying Your Health by Randall Fitzgerald (A Plume Book 2006)

The Illustrated Herb Encyclopedia: A Complete Culinary, Cosmetic, Medicinal, And Ornamental Guide to Herbs, by Kathi Keville (Mallard Press 1991). Pp 33

The Way of Ayurvedic Herbs, by Karta Purkh, Singh Khalasa, and Michael Tierra (Lotus Press, 2008, pp 89, 162

The illustrated Guide to Professional Hair Care and Hairstyles by Nicky Pope(South Water 2012) pp 10—11

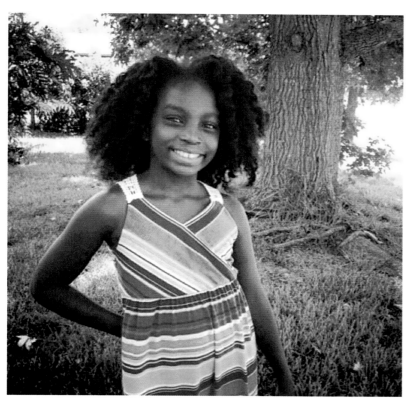

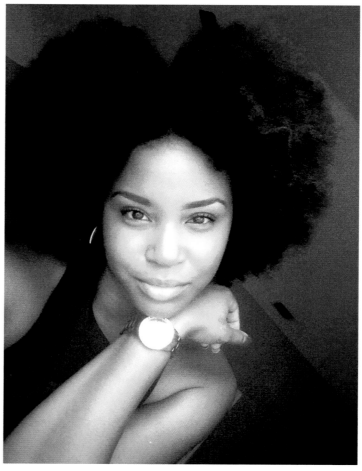

ABOUT THE BOOK

Nubia's Guide to Going Natural provides alternatives to hair care. To optimize your awareness of hair care, different oils, shampoos, hair care techniques, healthy benefits, and more are included in this publication.

This book does not promote any particular hair care products. The focus is to improve your overall wellbeing. Organic hair care guides you toward a successful, healthy transition. Going natural isn't limited to any specific race, sex, or gender. This book offers universal solutions to natural hair care. Adopt a chemical free way of life and embrace the natural approach. Natural hair is unprocessed hair and requires minimal chemicals to reserve its natural state.

As you begin your transition journey explore different hair types and learn from people who have a similar hair type. Nubia's favorite vloggers are included to guide you. The bloggers share step by step tutorials for successful hair styling. Stay tuned and join me under Natural Nubian on Facebook.

Printed in the United States
By Bookmasters